The Breathing Book

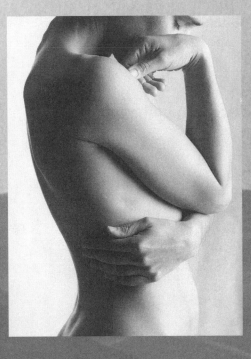

ILLUSTRATIONS BY

STEPHEN CROWE

An Owl Book

Henry Holt and Company
New York

The Breathing Book

~

Good Health and Vitality

Through

Essential Breath Work

~

DONNA FARHI

For Ray Worring,
who reached out and brought me
back to life

Owl Books
Henry Holt and Company, LLC.
Publishers since 1866
175 Fifth Avenue
New York, New York 10010
www.henryholt.com

An Owl Book® and ⊞® are registered trademarks
of Henry Holt and Company, LLC.

Library of Congress Cataloging-in-Publication Data
The breathing book: good health and vitality through essential breath work / Donna Farhi.
"An Owl book."
ISBN-13: 978-0-8050-4297-9
ISBN-10: 0-8050-4297-0
1. Breathing exercises. I. Title.
RA782.F37   1996   96–13286
613'.192   CIP

Henry Holt books are available for special promotions
and premiums. For details contact: Director, Special Markets.

First Edition 1996

DESIGNED BY KATE NICHOLS

Nature photographs by Bruce Young, Christchurch, N.Z.
Photographs by Fred Stimson, San Francisco
Illustrations by Stephen Crowe

Printed in the United States of America
15   17   19   20   18   16

A CAUTION

This book is not a prescription for health problems or a replacement for necessary medical treatment. If any of the inquiries or exercises causes you discomfort or shortness of breath, do not persist. Shortness of breath can be a sign that you are trying too hard to do the exercises, but it could also be an indication of a more serious health problem. Some health conditions and diseases are accompanied by changes in the quality and rate of breathing (for example, hyperventilation is a common compensation for and symptom of kidney disease). If you are at all in doubt, seek the advice of your health practitioner.

Contents

III: The Anatomy of Breathing 47

IV: Catching Your Breath 69

Part Two: Opening to the Breath

V: Room to Breathe   107

VI: Breathing Deeper   145

Practice Guides   *199*

Introduction

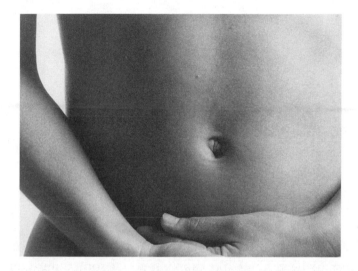

An immortal said, "To learn the way of the Tao is like recalling what you have eaten in the morning. It is not impossible to do. To treasure breath is like loving your face and your eyes. It has never been unattainable."

—MASTER GREAT NOTHING OF SUNG-SHAN,
TAOIST CANON ON BREATHING

How to Use This Book

$\mathcal{B}$reathing is not an intellectual activity. It may therefore seem strange at first to be reading and thinking about something you do all the time. From the very first breath at birth till the last whisper of breath leaves our bodies at death, breathing is something the body knows how to do for our basic survival. Right now as you read this book your body is breathing you and tonight when you go to bed your breath will flow in and out without any thought on your part. This automatic breath allows you to survive, but when you unconsciously hold or restrict your breath through habit, the breath that once so conveniently breathed you becomes *automatically restricted and distorted*. This unconsciously altered breath allows you to survive but it does not allow you to thrive. Thus, to reclaim what has always been a part of you requires your conscious awareness and participation.

Breathing affects your respiratory, cardiovascular, neurological, gastrointestinal, muscular, and psychic systems and also has a general effect on your sleep, your memory, your energy level, and your concentration. Everything you do, the pace you keep, the feelings you have, and the choices you make are influenced by the rhythmic metronome of your breath. As you are challenged, as we all are today, with increasing levels of psychological, physical, and biological stress, the internal metronome that determines the quality and state of your breathing and health may be set at faster and faster speeds. You may have the feeling that your life has become like that of a hamster—endlessly running on a little wheel, with no way to stop and get off. You say you feel "stressed out" or "burned out," and the tension and anxiety that accompanies that all-too-familiar state of over-load seems to be undermining your genuine desire to take care of yourself. You may remember a time when you were full of energy, and wonder where that time went and how you can recover it. In looking for a solution it is easy to get caught up in details, in theories, and in complicated strategies, for we very seldom explore the easiest and most fundamental concepts. The process of breathing lies at the center of every action and reaction we make or have and so by returning to it we go to the core of the stress response. By refining and improving the quality of our breathing we can feel its positive impact on all aspects of our being.

Today, Western medical and scientific studies are proving again and again what the Eastern health traditions have known for centuries: when we breathe well, we create the optimum conditions for health and well-being. And when we don't, we lay the foundation for illnesses such as heart disease and high blood pressure. The ancients would roll their eyes that it has taken us this long to see the obvious. We can now take comfort in the knowledge that most modern scientific and medical research supports the belief that proper breathing is a cornerstone to our well-being.

When you were born your whole body breathed. Every cell quivered with the vitality of the breath. Every bone, muscle, and organ moved with every breath. Every nerve was energized by it, every blood cell carried it, and every moment took as its meter the phrasing of your breath. Today, most of us have forgotten what it feels like to breathe fully and wholly with the vitality of the newborn infant. We have forgotten this but we have not lost it. In reclaiming the fullness of our breathing we also reclaim many other dimensions of our lives.

To remember something forgotten requires many steps. Often the path to recovery is circuitous. To make these steps more direct it helps to become familiar with our bodies and to know how they work. At school we were taught mathematics, reading, and the geography of the world, but few of us were taught much about the geographical mapping of the home we live in—our bodies. So this book is a fresh introduction to a place you've lived all your life but might not have noticed.

Throughout this book there are anatomical descriptions and exercises that act as signposts on the journey. But that's all they are because naming your breathing muscles cannot give you a direct experience of them. Use the poems, drawings, images, and inquiries as a way of entering the experience of your breathing more deeply. Imagine that you are becoming familiar with your body in the same way that you might come to know the layout of a new house, by walking through the same rooms and hallways over and over again. Keep looking and sensing from as many different perspectives so that gradually a multidimensional picture comes into focus. Knowing *where* you are directing your awareness and *what* you are directing your awareness upon makes the investigation more enriching. You will know the process is well underway when you begin to feel "at home" in your body.

It would be a mistake to approach this book as another "how-to-do" book. To do so would be only a repetition of how most of us have approached life in the past: trying hard, controlling, grasping . . . we are all too painfully aware of the failure of these strategies. Breathing fully is not a matter of adding anything, of acquiring some new technique, or of striving to improve oneself. Discovering the naturalness of our breaths has to do with uncovering or removing the obstacles that we have constructed to the breath, both consciously and unconsciously. In this sense, this book is a guide to a process of deconstruction, of unlearning and clearing away. It is a "how-to-undo" book.

This book will become a valuable guide to uncovering your breath only if you become actively involved with the questions, inquiries, and exercises. Take the time to pause throughout each chapter and use the questions, inquiries, and guided relaxations to embody the information step by step. Don't try to do too much in one session or even in one day. You may also want to repeat, as I do, a particular inquiry for many weeks or even months if you found it helpful. As you progress to more advanced inquiries it can be enlightening to return to the simpler ones to gauge how your awareness of your breathing has deepened.

Whether you are a psychotherapist wanting to add a somatic focus to your work, an athlete wanting to improve performance, a meditator, a business professional overcome by anxiety and stress, or someone who has simply noticed that his breathing is habitually shallow, this book can be an invaluable tool toward improving your breathing and well-being. I encourage you to use this book in an active way. It is your full interaction and participation with this information that will literally breathe life into it. Enjoy!

Part One

~

Fundamentals

I
The Essential Breath

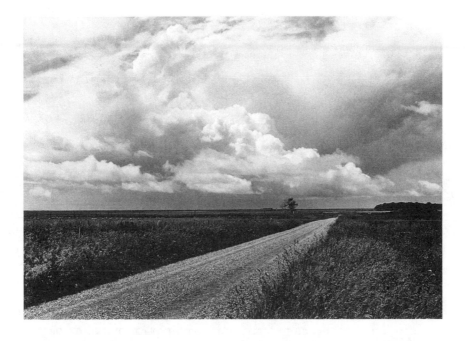

First of all the twinkling stars vibrated, but remained motionless in space, then all the celestial globes were united into one series of movements. . . . Firmament and planets both disappeared, but the mighty breath which gives life to all things and in which all is bound up remained.

—VINCENT VAN GOGH

What Is the Essential Breath?

*E*very day young children come to play in the sand at the beach where I live. They dance and spin, sing and shout, running wildly through the dunes and into the frothing surf, seemingly oblivious to the cold water and wind. Their aliveness is the envy of all the adults who stolidly tread the shore, amazed and exhausted by the relentless nature of the children's energy.

Most of us remember the exuberance of our own early youth when we breathed with relaxed open bellies and as a result had an almost limitless supply of energy. Then we began to learn and develop poor breathing patterns. Now, as adults we find ourselves looking for ways to reawaken this experience of aliveness—frequently turning to artificial uppers such as caffeine, sugar, nicotine, alcohol, or expensive megadoses of vitamins and herbs. Feeling the agitation that results from artificial stimulants we may resort to tranquilizers and sleeping pills to quell our growing unease, and thus begin a roller coaster of ups and downs. Or we subsist on the excitement of one fleeting moment after another using sex or our obsession with work and material possessions to momentarily ignite us. We have a sneaking suspicion that we could feel better, more energetic, more at peace, and that something, something not quite definable, is missing from our lives. Curiously the answer to recovering this dynamic vitality lies intrinsically within us—in the unconditioned breath that we had as a child.

Breathing is the most readily accessible resource you have for creating and sustaining your vital energy. Tapping this resource involves a process of unleashing the potent elixir of what I call the "essential" breath. This is the breath you breathed as a young child. Most of us have lost a connection with this breath and so have lost a connection with a natural way of being and our own natural energy resource. Opening the doors to this life force involves rediscovering the virgin nature of the breath.

Breathing is one of the simplest things in the world. We breathe in, we breathe out. When we breathe with real freedom, we neither grasp for or hold on to the breath. No effort is required to pull the breath in or to push the breath out. Given the simplicity of breathing one would think it was the easiest thing to do in the world. However, if it were truly so easy there would be few unhappy or unhealthy people in the world. To become a welcome vessel for the breath is to live life without trying to control, grasp, or push away. And how easy is this? The process of breathing is the most accurate metaphor we have for the way that we personally approach life, how we live our lives, and how we react to the inevitable changes that life brings us.

> A tree growing out of the ground is as wonderful today as it ever was. It does not need to adopt new and startling methods.
>
> —ROBERT HENRI

Throughout time the process of breathing was always considered inseparable from our health, consciousness, and spirit, and it is only recently that we have reduced breathing to a mere respiratory exchange of carbon dioxide and oxygen. In Greek, *psyche pneuma* meant breath/soul/air/spirit. In Latin, *anima spiritus,* breath/soul. In Japanese, *ki,* air/spirit; and in Sanskrit, *prana* connoted a resonant life force that is at no time more apparent to us than when that force is extinguished at the moment of death. In Chinese the character for "breath" (*hsi*) is made up of three characters that mean "of the conscious self or heart." The breath was seen as a force that ran through mind, body, and spirit like a river running through a dry valley giving sustenance to everything in its course.

Today, our intuition about the potential power of the breath is firmly embedded in the very structure of our language. We speak about the breath in common, everyday expressions but it rarely occurs to us to associate this with our immediate bodily experience. We say that we need "a breath of fresh air," "You take my breath away," "I couldn't catch my breath," or "I waited with bated breath." Or exclaim that something was "simply breathtaking!" We complain of someone "breathing down our neck" and needing "room to breathe," "breathing a sigh of relief," or "taking a breather." We tell our friends "not to breathe a word," and we complain about being "out of breath." And yet few of us, when faced with fatigue, illness, or anxiety, look to our breath as a possible source for regeneration. Because it is right under our noses, the significance of this ever renewable source of energy has escaped our attention.

Most people are not aware that they breathe poorly. Fewer still are aware of the consequences of restricting this central life process. From headaches to heart disease and a vast array of common maladies in between, breathing badly takes its secret toll. Most significantly, very few people understand the ways in which they restrict and distort their breathing. Habitually breathing high into the chest, breathing too fast, and breathing shallowly are epidemic today. And one does not need the trained eye of a respiratory specialist to recognize these patterns in ourselves and in others. A casual glance of any city street will reveal the extent to which tight belts, tight bodies, and tight schedules are literally taking our breath away.

Correlations between breathing and the state of our body and mind have been made for thousands of years in ancient Taoism, in Yogic scriptures, and in the medical practices of India (Ayurveda), Tibet, and China. More recently, countless scientific studies have supported this ancient wisdom, linking effortless breathing with the mitigation of some of our most insidious modern health problems. Breath therapy, sometimes combined with other healing practices such as biofeedback or yoga, has been found to alleviate (and sometimes cure) migraine headaches,[1] chronic pain conditions,[2] hypertension (high blood pressure),[3] epilepsy,[4] asthma,[5] panic attacks, and hyperventilation syndrome,[6] as well as coronary heart disease.[7] A recent study by Suzanne Woodward and Robert Freedman showed that slow, deep breathing *alone* will result in a significant reduction in menopausal hot flashes.[8] In a pilot study prior to their own research, progressive muscle relaxation exercises and slow, deep breathing reduced the incidence of hot flashes by an impressive 50 percent.[9]

Breathing techniques are also being used to help those with life-threatening illnesses enter a meditative state and calm the terror that often accompanies illness and death. Two of the major proponents of "comeditation" or "cross breathing," Richard Boerstler and Hulen Kornfeld, have been teaching this ancient Tibetan technique at hospitals and medical schools throughout the United States. (See Resources for more information.) According to Patricia A. Norris, Ph.D., clinical director of the Menninger Clinic's Biofeedback and Psychophysiology Center, her staff has been using comeditation since it was introduced to them in 1987 by Boerstler and Kornfeld. As Norris enthusiastically relates, "We use it for people in severe pain or with serious neuromuscular disorders. It is especially helpful for people who are anxious and unable to slow their breathing. The recipients say they have never felt so relaxed. We find it eases anxiety, tension, and pain. We also teach it to family members, who are happy to have something that allows them to feel helpful, connected, and at one with the patient."[10]

Relaxation research shows that breathing techniques can help ward off disease by making people less susceptible to viruses and by lowering blood pressure and cholesterol levels. When we breathe in a relaxed fashion we move from a destructive metabolic state to a constructive one. This shift from operating in a chronic stress mode to a mode of relaxed alertness can affect the synthesis of protein, fat, and carbohydrates, increase the production of cells for immune system activation, promote bone repair and growth, as well as enhance the cellular, hormonal, and psychological processes.[11]

We experience the benefits of these chemical, cellular, and neurological changes on a more subjective level in the way we feel and think. People who practice open breathing through healing arts such as tai chi, yoga, or mindful meditation, are rewarded not only with optimal health; they also seem to have a different relationship to life's stresses. They are able to remain calm and centered in the midst of seeming chaos. We speak about such people as being grounded, centered, and having "presence of mind." Perhaps the most universal experience of my own breath work students is their new-found ability to handle tough situations with an ease that previously seemed illusive. Just as each breath arises with its own uniqueness, they have learned to open to each moment as new and different, and as a result, are finding new solutions to tenacious problems. As their minds become clearer and their emotions become more balanced through calm and regular breathing, they are creating a life that is conducive to health, well-being, and a sense of inner peace. And not so surprisingly, I notice that people who do breathing practices act and appear much younger than their chronological age.

Perceiving the essential breath and becoming conscious of its natural state is very different than controlling or manipulating the breath through quick techniques and exercises. At first it may be difficult to understand this seemingly subtle point but it is a crucial distinction. The breath is one of the many unconscious processes in the body that can be voluntarily controlled. However, recovering the extraordinary flexibility that is the hallmark of free breathing cannot be achieved by force or will alone. Breathing techniques can be very powerful but rarely do artificial means of controlling and manipulating the breath provide long-term, positive benefits.

Our breath has been with us since birth, but as we grew we began to unconsciously alter and interfere with the free expression of the breath. Adding artificial or contrived methods of breathing may only serve to further obscure the process of awakening this natural breath. We do not need to create some other breath. Instead, we should focus our efforts in such a way as to seduce our dormant breath out of hiding. What is required is not a new, artificial way of breathing that lasts as long as our stunningly brief attention span, but to return to a way of breathing that can be calm and regular, flexible and spontaneous. This essential breath is always available to support whatever we do, whether we are running a marathon or running a business. Integrated breathing can be the cornerstone for all other human movement patterns and processes, allowing us to be confidently engaged in the world.

> What's the nature of the place? The proper approach to any kind of land use begins with that question. What is the nature of this place? And then: What will nature permit me to do here? . . . that way of thinking continues in the work of some modern agriculturalists . . . whose approach is to ask what the nature of the place is, what nature would be doing here if left alone. What will nature permit me to do here without damage to herself or to me? What will nature help me to do here?
>
> —WENDELL BERRY,
> *FIELD OBSERVATIONS*

The Breath Connection

Respiration is primarily regulated by involuntary controls through the central nervous system and so our bodies are breathing us automatically day and night. Controlled through the autonomic nervous system we don't have to think about breathing, it just happens . . . or does it? You might notice that your breathing is habitually shallow or that you sigh all the time. You may notice that you habitually hold your breath or restrict your breathing through particular strategies such as constantly tightening your belly. Perhaps you experience breathing as a great effort. Or you often feel out-of-breath. Maybe you don't notice your breathing at all but feel chronically tired, irritated, hurried, or anxious—so much so that these feelings cast a shadow over all your daily activities. When your breathing becomes unconsciously altered the autonomic part of your nervous system resets itself so that breathing becomes automatically *disordered* and automatically *restricted*. This resetting process will be explained in depth in later chapters. For now know that the deep level at which this process is taking place is the level we must enter to return the breath to its original flexibility. This is why attempting to alter the breath through mechanical exercises has a limited effectiveness, since we are not changing the underlying structures that support healthy breathing. On a deeper level, highly controlled breathing practices such as those employed in yogic *pranayama* can backfire because they can act to repress the underlying psychological fears and issues that are driving poor breathing habits in the first place.

> As for the proper inner breath, it is called the Embryonic breath. Since it is naturally inside you, you do not have to seek outside for it.
>
> —MASTER GREAT NOTHING OF SUNG-SHAN, *TAOIST CANON ON BREATHING*

At one end of the spectrum is the unconscious, involuntary breath; at the other end is breathing that is controlled and regulated by the will, such as the classic breathing exercises done by yogis. Between these two extremes lies the "essential" breath, a conscious flow that arises out of the depth of our being and dissolves effortlessly back into our core. It arises from a background that is still and silent and dissolves back into this same stillness. To access this essential breath, we must first be able to focus on and perceive our own breathing process; that is, we must make the unconscious conscious.

Recovering the essential nature of the breath is a rich and rewarding process for it is ourselves that we uncover. Right now, with very little effort, you can begin to experience the essential breath. Take a moment to feel the presence of this breath inside you.

～ INQUIRY ～

The Essential Breath

Sitting comfortably in your chair begin to notice your breathing without trying to alter it or make it in any way different. Just let your breath do what it will. Slowly begin to rest your attention on your exhalation and let your awareness travel down the length of an exhalation. Do this a number of times, enjoying the sensation of the breath effortlessly leaving the body. What do you find at the end of the exhalation? Did you feel the momentary pause that follows the end of the exhalation? This pause may be brief, a momentary hesitation, yet something very special happens in that pause. Don't try to make the pause happen or to extend it forcefully. Simply relax and let it happen. As you surrender to the restfulness in the pause you may find that it lengthens on its own accord. Trust that the next breath can arise out of the pause without you "grabbing" for it.

Within this pause there is no thought and no movement. You may experience it as a pregnant silence, much like the silence you feel when you enter a forest. The new breath arises out of this pause. The next moment arises out of this pause. The inhalation is born out of the stillness of the pause and the exhalation dissolves into it.

This pause is a well, a resource that is always available to you. Know that at any time when you feel tired or confused, hurried or overwhelmed, you can draw from this well for rest and replenishment simply by entering the pause at the end of the exhalation. Without anticipating or projecting the outcome of the next moment, can you wait and see what the next breath brings?

Untying the Breath

The challenge in uncovering and reawakening the essential breath is in learning to see how we interfere or block this natural process. All too often, we may unconsciously breathe so fast that we no longer allow for the resting pauses in the breath rhythm. We also may employ any number of conscious and unconscious restraints upon our breathing process so that the original balance of the process is masked. The inquiries in the following chapters are designed to gently remove these restrictions so that the essential breath is revealed. They are called inquiries rather than exercises because an exercise implies doing something repetitively or by rote, which is not at all the state of mind necessary for this investigation. Doing an exercise also assumes there is a set result we are trying to achieve, while there is not necessarily one correct answer or outcome to an inquiry.

In your eagerness to untie your breathing you may pull and tug on yourself, and in doing so unwittingly increase the tension in your breathing. If you can be patient during the inquiries you will find that the breath will magically open to you in the same way that a knot falls open when you play with it patiently. There is very little between you and the magic of this opening.

II
The Breath That Moves Us

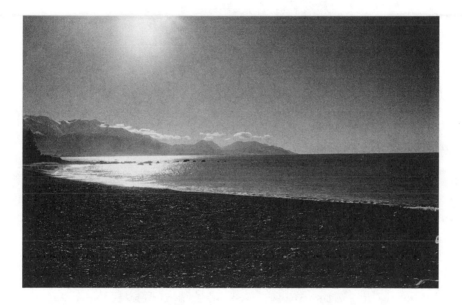

The great sea

Has sent me adrift

It moves me

As the weed in a great river

Earth and the great weather

Move me

Have carried me away

And move my inward parts with joy.

—UVAVNUK/ESKIMO

*O*ur breath is constantly rising and falling, ebbing and flowing, entering and leaving our bodies. Full body breathing is an extraordinary symphony of both powerful and subtle movements that massage our internal organs, oscillate our joints, and alternately tone and release all the muscles in the body. It is a full participation with life.

The fundamental nature of the breath is that, like life, it is constantly changing. The breath oscillates. It rocks us to and fro, fills and empties us, expands and condenses. One of the easiest ways to begin to perceive this natural flow of the breath is to learn to recognize the basic movements in the body that are present during breathing. Movement tells you where the breath is moving . . . and where it is not. Recognizing these movements is the first step in getting to know your breath.

When the challenges of life seem too great to handle, or things aren't going as smoothly as we planned, we may try to stop the natural flow of events by unconsciously restricting these movements. We stop our breath as a way of attempting to bring life under our command. Because there is such a strong tendency to restrict the movement of the breath, the second step in reclaiming the breath is to begin to notice how we are preventing the breath from entering and leaving the body freely. Neither step involves great effort or adding anything, but both require the cultivation of self-awareness or self-reflective consciousness.

The marriage of breath and movement is deep and abiding. It is a marriage that began with your very first breath at birth. The next time you have a chance to hold a newborn baby, notice how every single part of a child's body moves with his or her breathing. Your family cat may be an equally helpful role model.

Many of us feel ourselves disconnected from our bodies, often having no more familiarity with the physical frame that carries us than with a remote distant cousin. If you feel unfamiliar with your body it is only natural that in the beginning your perceptions will be vague and indistinct. You may have only a very general or diffuse sense of your breathing, but even this fleeting awareness is cause for celebration. Rest assured that it will not be long before your perception becomes more localized and refined. Your breath then will become like a friend you know well. The inquiries in this book take into account this natural progression of awareness and range from very simple to very subtle. Take the time to work with the simple ones before you move on.

Developing Breath Perception

The quality of attention that we bring to our investigation of the breath is crucial. The word *concentration* has come to be associated with the image of a pen gripped with white fingers or with fiercely furrowed brows. Given these misconceptions it is logical to think that if we try hard and especially if we try to breathe deeply, our breathing will be improved. Anyone who has tried these strategies knows that they do not work very well. In the following inquiries, instead of trying to grip your body with your awareness, let openness and patience be your guide. Instead of demanding results, inquire, feel, and sense. *The most important thing to remember in all these investigations is that there is no ideal in the process of perception.*

Our efforts to make the breath deeper may also be driven by all kinds of false and incorrect ideas about breathing, which will be discussed in detail in later chapters. The paradox of free breathing is that it is a result of deep relaxation, not of effort. Trying hard through pushing and striving does not help us open the breath. We may also have ideas based on what we were told as children (and as adults) as to what it means to breathe "deeply." If you are like most people, breathing deeply means to "sniff" the nostrils together, and to suck the breath in while pushing the chest out. Our drive to be productive together with our ideas about how we think we should breathe can be a major obstacle to recovering the naturalness of the breath.

If you find yourself labeling your perceptions—"Oh, this is a good way to breathe . . . this must mean I'm breathing wrong . . . I should be breathing more deeply . . . it's hopeless, I'll never get it right . . . ,"—you will most likely find it very difficult to receive them with an open mind. You might also be asking, "What *should* I feel?" Instead ask yourself what it is that you *do* feel, and you will be on the right path. Trust that if you let go of your preconceived ideas and expectations the vitality of the breath will emerge naturally.

Preparing for the Inquiries

I suggest that before beginning any of the inquiries and explorations in this book you remove restrictive clothing such as belts or bras. Loosen or unfasten any collars or cuffs and if possible change into a loose-fitting outfit. Undo any barrettes or ponytails that might press into your head or cause your head to tilt to one side. If you are wearing glasses or contact lenses you may want to remove them so your eyes can relax. Whenever possible, turn off the sound to the phone, close the door, and make sure the room is warm and the floor well padded with a rug or blanket. Let the members of your household know that you don't want to be disturbed. You might even want to cover yourself with a soft blanket so that your body can be completely relaxed. Although you want to be as relaxed as possible it's usually not a good idea to do your inquiries in bed since the body associates bed with sleeping. Take the time to prepare yourself and your surroundings so you'll get the most out of each session.

Although it's ideal to practice the inquiries in "hothouse" conditions where you have the least distractions, you can do most of the inquiries in this book in any work or public setting. Most of the reclining inquiries can be done sitting in a chair or standing up. You can maximize the benefits by taking discreet measures such as loosening your belt or taking off your glasses for a few minutes. I have done my breath work on airplanes, in buses, and while walking on city streets, without drawing any attention to myself. This can be a very powerful way to integrate breathing awareness into all your everyday activities.

In a number of the inquiries I suggest the optional use of a partner. While this can certainly be helpful, it is not at all necessary. All the inquiries can be done alone and you should not feel you are getting less out of your work if you do not have a friend to help you. Having a partner for some of the exercises can give you a more objective view of what you are doing and can also make it easier to focus in particular areas. Instructions for both options are included.

Checking In with Your Breath

To be able to compare and appreciate the changes that may occur both during and after a breathing inquiry, it's important to take a few moments beforehand to gauge the initial quality of your breathing. I call these observations breathing "check-ins," and they can be used not only before doing a breathing inquiry, but throughout the day as a way of gauging one's physical and psychological state. Generally when people start to observe the breath they immediately change it. Because of this tendency, in the beginning let your check-ins be brief. I call them "body glances." You need not collect a library of details during these check-ins. A general impression will suffice for now.

To get a general impression of your breathing take a moment now to sit and sense your breathing. As you ask yourself the following questions wait for your reactions to come through.

"Where do I feel my breathing?"

Can you feel where the movement of the breath originates? At first you may say that you feel nothing. But when you return to this question at the end of an inquiry you may find that your breathing feels deeper, fuller, or less effortful. Let whatever perceptions you have come through without editing or analyzing them. Don't discount small movements or seemingly insignificant perceptions. It's all significant. Do you feel particular areas of your body where the breath is more noticeable? Around your abdomen, chest, or nostrils? Throughout the rib cage? Do you notice your breathing around your shoulders or your breastbone?

"What does my breathing feel like?"

What is the quality of your breathing? Is it rough, labored, jerky, rhythmic? Does it feel smooth or mechanical? Take note of whatever words or images arise. You may want to record them for future reference.

Take the time to do a "body glance" before and after the other inquiries and movements. Now you are ready to start the first inquiry.

～ INQUIRY ～

The Marriage of Breath and Movement[1]

You'll Need

A chair

Purpose

This inquiry is designed to clarify the relationship between breath and movement. It can serve as a springboard for your own creative exploration.

Here's How

Sit on a hard chair so you can feel your pelvic bones in contact with the chair. Let the chest be balanced over the center of your belly. Place your hands on your thighs with the palms facing upward; gently stretch the hands so the fingers are softly extended but not tense. Then relax the hands and let the fingers curl inward so your palms form a slight hollow. Continue to rhythmically fold and unfold the hands. Continue for a few minutes in this way. Then begin to observe your breath. Do you notice any relationship between the movement of your hands and when you inhale and exhale?

Now extend this movement so that you open and turn out your arms and then relax and turn in your arms. Let the movement expand into your chest so that your chest opens as you gently extend the arms (Figure 1) and so that it settles and folds inwards as you turn the arms inwards. Let your entire spine come into the movement so that the whole body opens and closes like a sea anemone (Figure 2). Observe again how your breath is moving in response to the movement of the body. Let the movement get large and expansive. Feel how the breath changes as the movement grows larger and then gradually over a period of minutes let the movements get smaller and smaller until you are quiet and still. As you cease the large physical movements of the body and become quiet can you still feel the echo of the movement inside you like a pulse? Has your breath changed in any way?

The movement of the hands and arms stimulates the movement of the breath

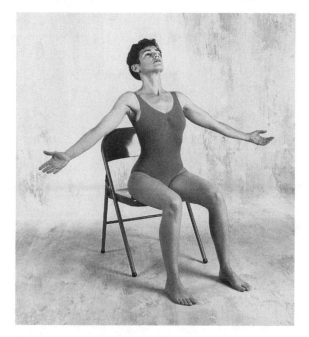

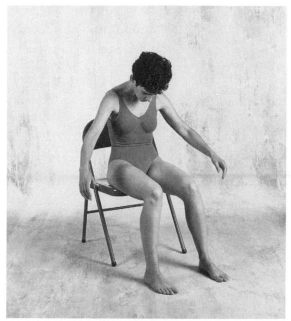

FIGURE 1

FIGURE 2

and determines the rhythm and the speed of the breath. As your breath deepens on its own accord, it may start to feel as if the breath is causing the movement. The inhalation asks the hands to unfold and the exhalation gently retrieves the fingers inward. Some people find this rhythm reversed, which is just fine. Notice your unique relationship with the breath. Is the breath causing the movement? Is the movement causing the breath? Each is inseparably entwined with the other.

Take a few moments to settle after completing this inquiry before doing a check-in with yourself. How has your perception of your breathing changed? You can use this simple exercise to "kick start" your breathing if it has become shallow or restricted. Even in the most public of places, opening and closing your hands will not draw attention to you.

When you are ready you may want to continue by learning the Effortless Rest position. This will be a starting position for many of the breath inquiries. Because it is effortless, this position allows you to focus completely on your breathing. It does have one disadvantage—it is so relaxing that you may drift off or even fall asleep. Sitting on a cushion or in a chair will increase attentiveness.

Experiment with the alternative positions that are described below, using the ones you find most comfortable and effective. Also feel free to change from one position to another during an inquiry.

～ INQUIRY ～

The Effortless Rest Position

You'll Need

> A warm, quiet room
> 1–2 blankets
> A bath towel or small pillow

Purpose

Finding a neutral relaxation position from which we can observe the breath is the starting point for most of the inquiries in this book. The objective is to find a balance between relaxation and attentiveness rather than unconscious slumber. The relaxation position acts as a base line from which we can venture forth and to which we can return. Take the time to find the positions that are most comfortable for you.

Here's How

This position will allow you to observe your breath and movement comfortably for up to 30 minutes. Begin by lying with your back on the floor. Bend your knees and place your feet hips-width apart. Experiment with the distance between your heels and your buttocks and the distance between the two feet until you find the place where the bones of the upper and lower legs rest like cards against each other with no effort. If you find your thighs tensing you have probably bent your legs too much. If your abdomen is tense your heels are probably too far away from your buttocks. Fold the bath towel to make a small pillow and place this under your head and neck so that the edge just grazes the top of the shoulders (Figure 3). Let yourself settle and with an audible exhalation

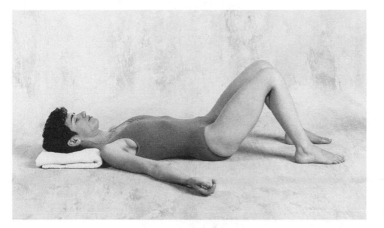

FIGURE 3

allow any distractions to fall away. Knowing that your worries and concerns, your responsibilities, and your difficulties will surely be waiting for you when the session is over, make an agreement with yourself to put them aside for this short period.

Alternative Relaxation Positions for the Inquiries

If you do not find the Effortless Rest Position comfortable, or you find it difficult to remain attentive while lying down, here are some possible alternatives. Feel free to explore and use these during the inquiries.

Sitting Cross-Legged (Figure 4) Place a cushion or a stack of blankets underneath your buttocks. Adjust the height until your knees lie below the level of your hips. This is important because if your knees are up in the air, the lower back will collapse backward, causing the front of the body to compress. This will constrict the diaphragm and make breathing difficult. If you like the feeling of attentiveness that accompanies sitting, but find it strains your back, try sitting with your back against a wall.

Kneeling (Figure 5) Place a small cushion or a folded blanket or towel between your sitting bones and your heels. This will make the position easier on your knees. Alternatively, if you have a meditation bench you can use that.

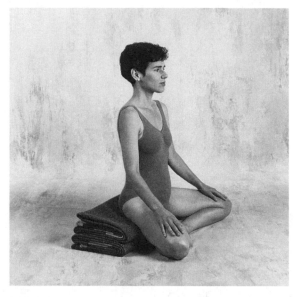

FIGURE 4

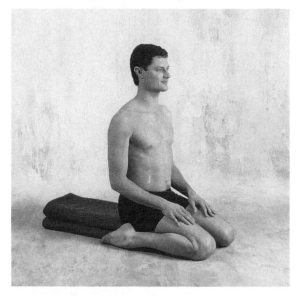

FIGURE 5

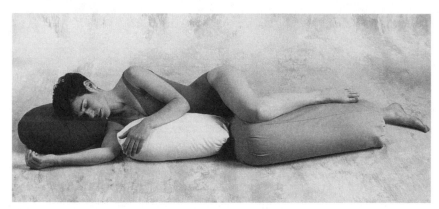

FIGURE 6

Side-Lying (Figure 6) Side-lying is especially comfortable for pregnant women and those with back pain. (Lying flat on the back is contraindicated after the third month of pregnancy because it may restrict the blood flow to the fetus.)

This side position can restrict your breathing on one side of the body, but for short periods of relaxation it can be a real boon. Try alternating sides between inquiries. When you lie on your side, place a pillow underneath your head so that your head and neck do not bend to one side but feel supported. Also place a pillow between your knees so that your back does not twist. If you are in the later stages of pregnancy it will be especially comforting to have a pillow in front of your chest so that you can drape your arm around it and a pillow behind you to support your back. Although it sounds cumbersome, my pregnant students relish this relaxation position because they can momentarily relinquish the extra weight of the baby.

Sitting on a Chair (Figure 7) If you are going to sit on a chair, find one that does not have wheels and that allows you to have both feet flat on the floor. A low stool is ideal. It is best to work sitting on the edge of the chair with your feet placed slightly wider than your hips so that your buttocks and the two feet form a stable tripod. If your back is very weak, try sitting with your back against the chair for support.

Child's Pose (Figure 8 shown with modifications) Some people find this position particularly helpful for feeling the movement of the breath in the belly and pelvic area. To get into it, start by kneeling and then gently fold forward until your head is resting on the floor in front of your knees and your arms are draped either side of your legs with the palms up. If you find this uncomfortable on your

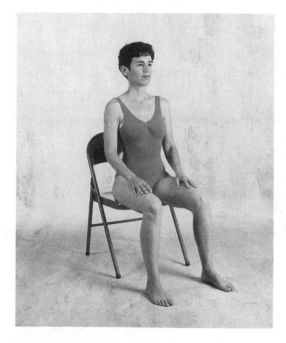

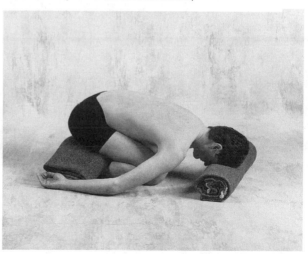

FIGURE 7

FIGURE 8 (shown with modifications)

knees, try putting a blanket in between your heels and your buttocks and a small pillow underneath your forehead.

Feel free to move from one position to another so that you are comfortable at all times. Now you are ready to begin.

Remember: Always precede your inquiries with a brief "check-in." Observe where you feel your breathing and the general quality of your breathing. This will help you to appreciate and contrast the changes that occur as a result of your breath work.

～ INQUIRY ～

How Do I Breathe?

You'll Need (5–10 minutes)

A note pad and pen
A partner (optional)

Purpose

The primary purpose of this inquiry is to gather more specific information than you might during a brief breath check-in. Do not breathe in a certain way or make your breath big and impressive. Simply notice your particular breathing style. It is helpful to enter the inquiry with curiosity and inquisitiveness rather than a desire to get it right. This is not a pass or fail exercise! Drop any ideas about how you think you should breathe. Watch for the judgmental mind that discounts small movements as insignificant or unimportant or the ambitious mind that jumps in to tell you to make your breath bigger or deeper, or labels your perceptions as good or bad in order to arrive at a conclusion. Acknowledge whatever you can feel and take special note of places where you can't sense any movement at all.

Here's How

You can do this inquiry alone or with an observing partner. The advantage of having a partner is that you can compare your impressions with the observations of your friend. For instance, you may think you breathe slowly, but your partner observes that you take twenty-two breaths a minute. Your partner can also guide you through the questions. If you are a helper in this inquiry be sure to give your partner lots of time between questions.

Start in the Effortless Rest position or any of the other sitting positions. Begin by resting one hand on your belly below the navel and one hand on the breast bone in the center of your chest.

Give yourself a minute or two to investigate each question.

- **Location of the Breath** Where is the movement of the breath most noticeable? In the lower part of my body or in the upper part? Once you sense this, let your hands come down by your sides about a foot away from your hips with the palms up.

- **Origin of the Breath** Just as an earthquake has an epicenter that scientists can locate, your breath has an epicenter, too. Where does the movement of the breath begin?

- **Frequency of the Breath** Is your breath fast or slow or somewhere in between? Count the number of breaths per minute or if possible have a friend count them for you. Twelve to fourteen breaths per minute is considered a "normal" rate.

- **Phrasing of the Breath** Is there a noticeable difference between the length of your inhalation and exhalation? Are they equal?

- **Texture of the Breath** Is the texture of your breath smooth and even or is it jerky and uneven?

- **Depth of the Breath** Does the breath feel deep or shallow? It might be quite appropriate for your breath to be quiet in the Effortless Rest position, so don't try to make your breathing more impressive during this question.

- **Quality of the Breath** If you could describe the quality of your breath what word or words would you use? Is it pneumatic, labored, billowing? . . . Let descriptive words or images arise without altering them in any way. When I first started to notice my breathing it felt as if my lungs were trapped like prisoners inside my rib cage and my breathing had the quality of being thick and dense. Do you have any images that you associate with your breathing?

Now completely relax and allow your body to melt into the floor. Focusing your attention on the breath takes energy, so take a few minutes now to let yourself rest before rolling over on your side and sitting up. You may want to record your observations in a small notebook or if you are doing the exercise with a friend, partner, or in a group you may want to tell each other what you noticed. If you are listening to someone else, refrain from analyzing or interpreting the information they present to you. It is particularly upsetting to have one's breathing psychologically interpreted. This kind of judgment can also undermine trust. The purpose of the inquiries at this stage is not to arrive at a conclusion but to get a general sense of how you breathe normally.

～ INQUIRY ～

Movements of the Breath

You'll Need (15 minutes)

A quiet place to lie down

Purpose

The purpose of this inquiry is to notice some of the body movements that occur spontaneously during relaxed, unrestricted breathing. Once you gain a better sense of how your body moves with your breath you can use this as foundation for all daily activities.

The movements indicated in this inquiry are presented from the experience of the author and the students who have participated in these exercises. They are merely suggestions and not definitive in any way. You may notice other movements and sensations and these observations are as important, if not more so, than my own suggestions.

Because your breathing may not be relaxed or spontaneous at this stage it is just as useful to be able to perceive where you don't feel movement. Make a note of the areas in your body that feel tense and contracted. Having this information can help you identify where you'll want to focus in chapter 5, "Room to Breathe."

Here's How

For this inquiry you'll begin in the Child's pose and shift into the Effortless Rest position. Also, you might want to repeat the inquiry in a sitting or standing position.

The Movement of the Abdomen

Close your eyes. Take a moment to mentally scan your entire body and become aware of what you have brought with you to the inquiry today. Then begin to gently focus your attention on your abdomen, the area from just underneath the tip of your sternum to just above your pubic bone. Notice how your abdomen moves as you breathe in and out. Feel the swelling and settling sensations on the inhalation and the exhalation. Do you sense any tightness or constriction in your belly? Do you tend to pull the abdomen inwards or upwards? If you are not sure whether you are holding tension in the belly, tense the abdomen for 7 seconds by pulling the muscles inward and then release. Do this a few times until you can feel the difference between tension and relaxation here.

Notice that the abdomen billows outward in all directions—up, to the sides, and into your back body on the inhalation. On the exhalation it retracts back but does not *contract*. The retraction has a tone and firmness without being rigid or hard. Remember that you don't have to make either the inhalation or the exhalation happen by pushing the abdomen in or out. Simply let the movements arise on their own accord.

The Movement of the Pelvic Floor

Now bring your attention to the floor of your pelvis—this is the space from the pubic bone in the front to your tailbone in the back and side to side from one sitting bone to the other (see illustration 15). Especially notice the space from the genitals to the anal area with the perineum in between. Check that you are not gripping the anus or tightening through the urinary or genital sphincter muscles. Also check around the base of the buttocks for any unnecessary holding. If you're not sure whether you are holding tension in these areas, contract the buttocks, anus, and pelvic floor for about 7 seconds and then let go. Repeat this action several times, until you can recognize the difference between tension and relaxation in these areas.

Notice how the pelvic floor moves when you breathe in and out. Can you feel any opening, broadening movements on the inhalation? Can you sense any condensing, toning movements on the exhalation? Feel how your anus opens when you breathe in and how it gently retracts on the exhalation phase of the breath. Notice that it opens and retracts without any effort on your part. Also detect how the genital area opens and swells as you inspire and how it slightly retracts as you expire. Women may notice how the walls of the vagina fan out and the opening of the vagina broadens on the inhalation and how the vagina tones and draws inwards on the exhalation. If you have difficulty feeling any or all of these movements, let your jaw fall open so that the breath comes in and out of the mouth, freely letting any sounds or sighs come. Ah! Sighing is a wonderful way to help loosen the breath and all the muscles that help us breathe. Imagine that you have a lightbulb in your pelvic floor and that as you breathe in the light glows and as you breathe out it dims.

Feel the relationship between the pelvic floor and the free movement of your abdomen. Notice how the abdomen feels when the anus opens and closes freely and how it feels if you pull the anus in and up. Sense into your belly again. As the abdomen expands, the pelvic floor also expands, and as the abdomen retracts, the pelvic floor also retracts. Now tense your abdomen and pull it in and up. Hold it in for a few cycles of your breath and feel how the movement in the pelvic floor has also ceased. Now slowly release your abdomen and feel how the floor of the pelvis responds.

The Movement of the Sacrum, Coccyx, and the Lumbar Spine

Now switch to the Effortless Rest position. Bring your awareness to your sacrum and coccyx as well as your lumbar spine. Your sacrum is the large triangular bone that anchors the lower back into the pelvis. The greater portion of your sacrum lies just above the crack of your buttocks. And your coccyx, or tailbone, attaches to the bottom of the sacrum. If you are lying on the floor, most of

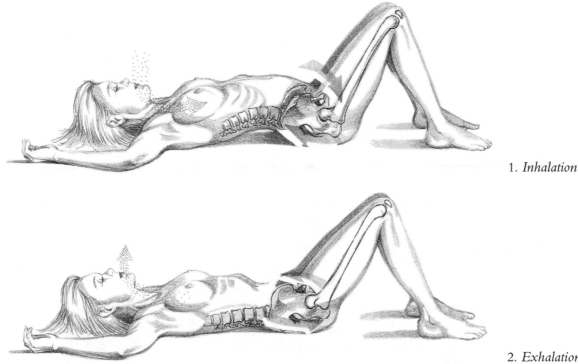

1. *Inhalation*

2. *Exhalation*

the weight of your pelvis will be on your sacrum. Begin to notice how your sacrum and coccyx move with your inhalation and exhalation. Can you feel how the tailbone arches away from the pubic bone on the inhalation? As the tailbone rocks to and fro, the sacrum also rocks on the floor. See if you can feel how the weight and pressure of your sacrum changes as you inhale and exhale. As you inhale, the whole pelvis tends to rock slightly into an arch so that the lower back moves away from the floor. As you exhale, the whole pelvis tends to rock so that the lower back flattens and lengthens on the ground. With each breath the lumbar spine gently extends, curving away from the floor and with each exhalation the lower back flattens toward the floor and elongates. Remember that these are small movements, more like a gentle swell than a strong mechanical action. If you contract your anus and pull the abdomen in, you will effectively prevent this wonderful movement from happening.

The movements you have just explored in the abdomen, pelvic floor, and in the sacrum, coccyx, and lower back are the basic building blocks of the natural breath. The roots of the essential breath lie in allowing these lower areas of the body to open and release fully.

Developmental Patterns—
Breathing the first pattern lays
the foundation for all the other
succeeding patterns. Wherever
the breathing is blocked in the
body, future patterns will be
blocked; wherever the breathing is free, the future patterns
will develop efficiently.

—BONNIE BAINBRIDGE COHEN,
SENSING, FEELING AND ACTION

Experiment with tensing and holding the abdomen, pelvic floor, and buttock muscles to see
what happens to your breath. How do you breathe
when you hold these muscles rigid? You can either
finish your inquiry here and take a rest or continue
up the body with the following inquiries.

The Movement of the Spinal Column

Once again feel how the tailbone and sacrum
tip back on inhalation and draw slightly under on
exhalation. This sets up a rhythm: Notice how
your lower back follows the movement of the
rocking pelvis, arching slightly on the in breath
and lengthening and flattening on the out breath.

Continue your observation along the entire spinal column. You might imagine that the spine is like a piece of driftwood and that as the wave of your breath
passes through the body, the vertebrae of the spine float up and down on top of
it. Are there parts of your spine where you feel this movement clearly? Are there
other segments that feel rigid?

The Movement of the Hips

Bring your awareness to rest on your hips. Can you feel how the swelling
motion of the inhalation causes the hip bones to broaden slightly out of the hip
sockets? If you press your hands against the sides of your hips you may be able to
sense the movement more clearly. You might also notice that as the abdomen fills
and empties and the pelvis rocks to and fro, the bones of the pelvis rotate around
the hip bones. Don't try to create these movements mechanically. Remember
that your intention is not to create a big impressive breath but to notice the natural movements.

If the muscles in your back and hips have become very tight over the years
through inactivity or injury, at first you may not be able to feel any of these
movements. Make a note of these areas and don't become discouraged. As you
progress with the exercises in chapter 5 your flexibility will dramatically increase,
allowing you to breathe and move more freely.

THE PELVIS

The two sides of the pelvis, called *ilium,* join to the sacrum in the back at the *sacroiliac* joints and at the *pubic symphysis* in the front. The word *pelvis* means basin and it acts as a container for the abdominal organs. The bones of the pelvis are united by heavy connective tissue and binding ligaments that in their healthy state have a degree of resilience. The spinal column is anchored to and arises out of the pelvis, and the thigh bones, or *femurs,* connect to the sides of the pelvis. So, when you breathe, move, and especially when you walk, there is a small but synchronized swinging motion between the sacrum and the ilium, between the pelvis and the hips, and between the pelvis and the spinal column. In people whose breathing and movement is whole and integrated there is a distinct rhythmic movement throughout the lower body during inhalation and exhalation.

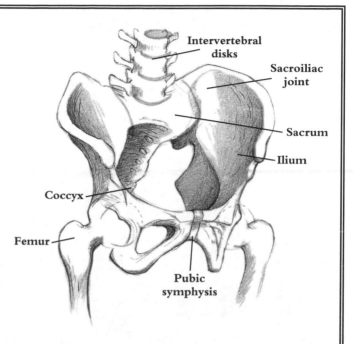

The Movement of the Shoulder Girdle and Arms

Sit or stand for this inquiry. Now bring your attention to your shoulders. As you inhale, see if you can feel the way the inhalation broadens the entire shoulder girdle. If you cross your arms in front of you and press on the outer shoulders with your hands (or do it on a partner) you may be able to feel this broadening movement. Feel the sensation spread from the breastbone through the collarbones to the shoulder sockets. You might also notice that the arms tend to rotate outward away from the center as you inhale and rotate inward toward the center as you exhale. If you find that your shoulders move predominantly up

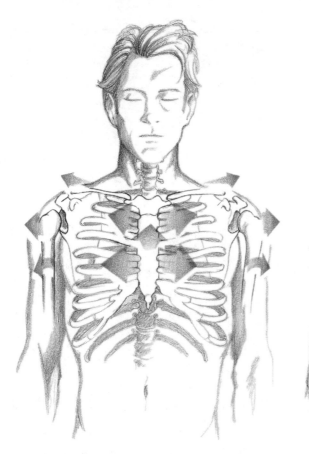

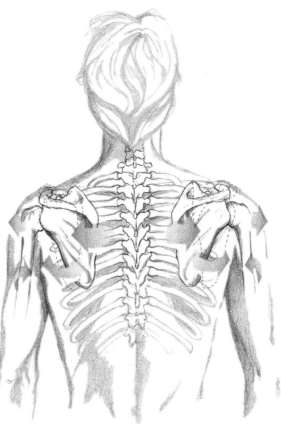

4. *The shoulder girdle and arms on inhalation.*
Front view

5. *The shoulder girdle and arms on inhalation.*
Back view

and down rather than horizontally, make a mental note of it. What other movements in your chest, shoulders, and arms can you feel as you breathe?

Now tighten and draw your abdomen inward and upward. Tighten and draw your pelvic floor inward and upward. Feel what happens to the movement of the breath in your upper body, neck, and shoulders as you restrict the movement in the lower body.

Full Body Breathing

Take any position you like for this last inquiry. To finish your breathing observation, imagine that your skin is like a knitted sheath that covers your entire body. As you inhale, feel how the strands of your sheath stretch and spread apart, creating space throughout the body. As you exhale, feel how the strands retract and the fiber becomes more dense and opaque. You can also use the pressure of your clothing against your skin as a way to observe the movement of the breath throughout the body. Enjoy the feeling of the whole body swelling and subsiding, filling and emptying. Take a few more moments to sense the places in your body that are opening with the breath. Are there any places in your body that don't participate in the dance of the breath? Make a mental note of these for later exploration. When you are ready, roll over on your side and rest until you feel ready to sit up. If you have been sitting on a chair or on the floor, hang forward over your thighs or lie on your back and relax for a few moments.

Important Observations

One of the things you may have noticed in the previous inquiries is that whenever you tightened the muscles in your lower body the breath was pulled up into your chest. You may have found your neck and shoulders and even your jaw tensing as you pulled your abdomen in, clenched the anus, or tightened the buttocks. When you restrict these natural movements the breath tends to become distorted. Instead of the abdomen swelling on the inhalation it draws inward and the upper chest rises. This is a common way for people to breathe when they are wearing restrictive clothing around their waists or if they are trying to look slimmer than they really are. This is called "chest breathing" (we'll look more closely at this and other breath holding patterns in chapter 4).

Under such circumstances, you tend to breathe with what is technically called the secondary respiratory muscles, muscles that were designed to come into play only during great exertion or in situations of oxygen deficit, such as after a sprint race. Instead of exaggerating your breathing in your chest, relax and allow all the muscles in the abdomen and pelvic floor to oscillate, which stimulates the deeper primary respiratory muscles to work to their full capacity.

Take a moment to note your observations during this inquiry. Also have a look now at the full body illustration showing a simplified version of some of the movements that occur during breathing.

Feeling the movements of the breath in a reclining relaxation position is helpful, but unfortunately we can't go through life this way. Being able to maintain your awareness of and allow these movements in everyday activities is a crucial step in maintaining full breathing at all times. In the next inquiries you'll

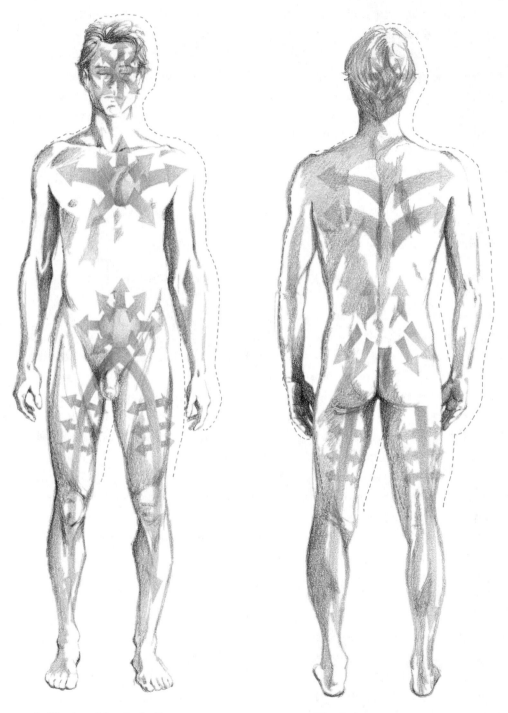

6. *The breathing body. Front*   7. *The breathing body. Back*

explore some common, everyday positions. As you assume these stances throughout the day continue to tune in to your breathing.

Squatting

Come to a squatting position with the arms extended in front of you for support (Figure 9). If your heels do not comfortably reach the ground, support them with a folded blanket. You also can do this inquiry sitting on the edge of a hard chair with your legs wide enough apart so that you can hang forward with your arms draped around the outsides of your thighs (Figure 10). Let your head relax forward so that the weight comes a little more onto your hands than on your feet. Check that you are allowing your abdomen to release freely with your breath and that you are not unconsciously gripping through the pelvic floor. Now look back between your legs at your crotch. Watch the movement of your pelvis as you breathe. Can you see the pelvis lift slightly up and back as you breathe in? Notice how the pelvis retracts back and down with the exhalation. Sense into your spine and see if you can feel how your lower back oscillates with the incoming and outgoing breath.

This wonderful movement of the pelvis rocking around the hips keeps the hip joints lubricated and the muscles there strong and flexible. These movements

FIGURE 9

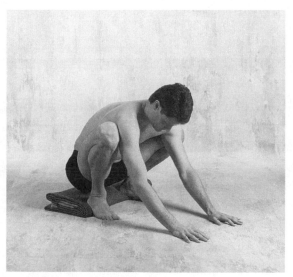

FIGURE 10

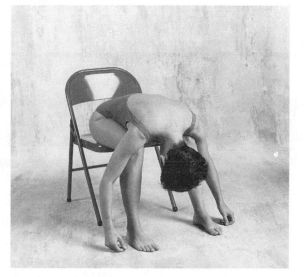

also keep the spine supple by keeping the circulation open and alternately toning and releasing the back muscles. Try tightening your abdomen and closing the anal sphincter muscles to see how this affects the movement in your pelvis and lower back. Experiment until you can feel the relationship between what you do with the muscles in the lower body and your breathing.

Sitting

Sit in a kneeling position or in any other comfortable sitting position. As you sit, have you already started to hold your belly in and pull up through the pelvic floor? Relax and observe your tailbone move forward and backward as you breathe in and out. See if you can feel any of the movements you noticed while lying on the floor in the earlier exercises. In your attempt to sit "properly," are you holding the body stiff against the fluid motion of the breath? When you breathe freely, there will be moments where the spine is slightly concave (arched) and less supported by the abdomen, and moments where the spine is slightly convex (rounded) and more supported by the abdomen. Again, these are small movements so don't discount what you feel because it does not appear large or impressive. This normal fluctuation massages all the internal organs and muscles, bringing fresh regenerative fluid and nutrition as well as removing depleted blood and waste products. If you sit for long periods of time, either working at a computer or for meditation, you may find that sitting in this fluid way prevents the tension and stiffness that many people experience when they attempt to sit "still."

Hanging Forward

Stand with your feet hips-width apart, knees *generously* bent. Bend your torso forward over your thighs. If you find the stretching sensations at the back of your legs so uncomfortable as to be distracting, you may want to do this exercise from your chair (see Figure 10). As you exhale, allow the weight of your breath to drop through the torso so the spinal column begins to elongate. Feel how the entire torso lifts and retracts slightly away from the floor as you breathe in, and then releases downward as you breathe out. Don't pull the torso downward against the natural rising movement of your inhalation. Allow your shoulder blades to rise on the inhalation and to drop with the exhalation and continue that release down the length of the arm. If you can't perceive any movement, try breathing through your mouth, sighing deeply as you exhale. Mouth breathing will create a less controlled breath and exaggerate the movements of the body, making them easier to observe. Finish up by checking for any holding at the base of the skull. This natural oscillation of the whole body releases deep held tensions and can be just as soothing and comforting to an adult as rocking is to a baby.

Remember that there is really nothing that you can *do* to make these movements happen—you can only *undo* or disengage from effort, so the breath can move freely through you.

If you are sitting in a chair, press down through your feet to come up, rolling up through your spine, so that your head is the last part of you to come upright. If you are hanging forward over your legs, come up in the same fashion, finishing in an upright standing position.

Standing Fluidly

As you stand, check your pelvic floor. You may be surprised to discover that you have automatically contracted your anus and lifted up through your belly in order to stand up straight. You may also notice that you tend to automatically hold your abdomen in when you stand. If this is true for you, exaggerate this action and observe how the energy shifts in your body. Can you feel tension increasing in your head, neck, and shoulders? Are you breathing more in your upper chest and neck?

Now allow your anus to open freely as you breathe in. Release the base of your buttocks down toward your heels and, instead of pulling your tailbone under, let the weight of your exhalation drop down through the tailbone. Allow the belly to be full and soft. Notice if tension decreases in your shoulders, neck, and head as you breathe lower in the body. Does standing like this make you feel more connected to the ground underneath you? Do you sense that you have "both feet on the ground" instead of "your head in the clouds" when you allow the weight of your pelvis to release into your legs?

Allow your knees to relax so that they are neither bent nor locked, but feel fluid underneath you. Can you detect any movement in your legs as you stand? Can you feel any movements in your shoulders and arms?

If you noticed that you tend to hold tension through your abdomen, buttocks, and pelvic floor when you stand, you may want to ask yourself this question: When did I first notice myself holding in my belly? Young children allow their bellies to protrude when they breathe, so restricting the belly is learned behavior. See if you can locate a period in time, and any particular situation, in which you found yourself holding in your abdomen. For instance, I remember getting a very strong message from a ballet teacher who, after stopping the class to increase the dramatic impact of her pronouncement, pointed to my relaxed belly and said, "*That* is the most disgusting thing I have ever seen!" I remember being particularly careful from that day on to keep my belly pulled in at all times. How does standing with your belly pulled in make you feel? How do you feel when you allow your belly to soften as you stand and to move freely with the breath? Let any images and thoughts arise freely without editing them. You may want to make a mental or written note of these thoughts and images, or if you are doing these inquiries with a friend, partner, or group, share what you observed.

～ INQUIRY ～

Where Do I Breathe?

You'll Need (30 minutes)

A partner (optional)
A soft mat or blanket to lie on
A folded towel
Quiet place where you will not be disturbed for 30 minutes

Purpose

The purpose of this inquiry is to become more aware of where you breathe. Through the help of a partner you can focus your attention completely on your breath, allowing your partner's touch to help you direct your awareness into specific areas. Although this inquiry can be done without the help of a partner, it is very nice to be able to relax completely while focusing awareness on your breath. If you want to work alone, just place your hands on your body, using gentle but firm pressure. The amount of pressure you would use to press a stamp onto an envelope is about right.

Note for helpers: In his research on breath retraining, Dr. Erik Peper of San Francisco State University has discovered that the most effective way for people to learn to breathe well is through modeling of the correct action by a skilled therapist or coach.[2] This method was the only one that significantly raised inhalation volume and lowered respiration rate. He also found that "emotions (and thus breathing styles) are contagious."[3] Our common sense tells us that people's energetic and emotional states affect us, so when you work with your friend be aware of your own breathing. Although you are probably not a trained therapist, it will help greatly for you to breathe into the same parts of your own body that you are touching on your partner. It can also help to breathe with your partner and encourage slower breathing by lengthening your own exhalation in synchrony with your partner.

Here's How

Lie down on a soft surface in the Effortless Rest position and place your folded towel underneath your head and neck. The helping partner can sit cross-legged (or in any comfortable position) at your head looking toward your feet. Take a few moments to adjust both your positions so that you won't be distracted.

Place one hand on your belly slightly above your navel and one hand on your chest near the top of your breastbone. Begin to notice how your breath is rising and falling under your hands. Your friend should take this time to observe your breath pattern. As you investigate the following questions, remember there is no right or wrong answer. Be inquisitive and withhold any judgments you may have about your breathing until later.

Without altering your breath, does one hand rise more than the other? Do you feel more movement in your chest or in your belly? Does one hand rise before the other or does the breath arise in both places at the same time? When you have a good idea of how you are breathing, let both your arms come down beside you, about a foot away from your hips with the palms turned up. This will cue your partner to begin assisting you. If your partner applies the wrong amount of pressure with her hands quietly let her know, but try to keep verbal interactions to a bare minimum so you can focus on your physical sensations.

Your helper is going to place her hands on different parts of your body. Alternatively you can use your own hands, pressing gently but firmly in each area. Wherever you touch, allow your breathing to emanate from that place. Rather than lifting the body mechanically, let your breathing be like a conversation with your own or your partner's hands. As you feel pressure on these different areas

FEELING BAD IN ORDER TO LOOK GOOD

We live in a time when there is an extreme obsession with looking trim, fit, and most important, young. This obsession is artificially created by industries that stand to gain from our cultivated insecurities. We are bombarded with the propaganda of the body beautiful (most models are thinner than 95 percent of the female population), believing that what we see is normal, and that we, in comparison, fall horribly short of these standards. In truth, images in women's magazines rarely go untouched or unaltered so that we now have no idea what a normal forty-year-old looks like because she has been been nose-jobbed, teeth-capped, collagen-enhanced, and air-brushed to look like a thirty-year-old princess. Men too are feeling the pressure of the advertising images—the washboard stomach is now the main focus of the "hard" muscular man. Young boys are almost on par with girls for unnecessary dieting, and cosmetic surgery for men is becoming commonplace. As a result we have a $33 billion a year diet industry, a $20 billion cosmetic industry, and a flourishing $300 million (and counting) cosmetic surgery industry.

We are being indoctrinated at a young age. In a survey of 494 middle-class school girls in San Francisco, 81 percent of the ten-year-olds were already dieters. By the time girls leave high school over 75 percent will feel extreme dissatisfaction with the weight and shape of their bodies, although few are actually overweight.

There are a plethora of statistics that tell us about the extent and economics of this mass hallucination, but they rarely tell us how we feel as a result. Underlying these figures, however, is the undeniable truth that we are willing to feel bad in order to look good. We are willing to walk around in a state of semi-asphyxiation, holding our bellies in with belts, zippers, and clothes two sizes too small, in order to cast the illusion of being youthful and fit. I recently worked with a woman suffering from severe panic attacks. She found that she could prevent and alleviate the symptoms of her attacks through full abdominal breathing but eschewed the idea of wearing clothes that allow for this because it was not, as she put it, "in keeping with her public image." She preferred to stay on debilitating and addictive medication rather than let herself breathe. It is not necessary to feel bad to look good. We may, however, have to change our definition of what "looking good" means.

If you wish to have a breathing body, a body filled with true energy and vitality, it will be necessary to reinvent yourself with your own definition of beauty. I am always amazed at how wonderful men and women look when they are comfortable in their bodies, regardless of the shape or size, and how even the most classically beautiful people appear unattractive when they are constricting (or have an obvious loathing for) their bodies. When you allow your body to breathe freely you will exude an air of confidence and ease so that your real beauty—who you are—can shine through. What makes you feel good can also make you look good.

TWO MYTHS ABOUT YOUR BELLY

Relaxing Your Belly Will Make It Bigger

There is a strong belief system in Western countries that constantly holding in the belly keeps the abdominal muscles strong. This belief rides in tandem with the notion that a pulled in abdomen looks better. A contemporary women's magazine featuring a truncated figure in "panty slimmers" lingerie, boasts that wearing a girdle will "target your tummy to control you where you need it most" and asks us to "think of it as a beautiful alternative to holding your breath." But we don't need panty slimmers. Most of us are already wearing a self-imposed psychic girdle most of the time that is far more damaging and powerful than any girdle—we walk around with our stomachs held in and we don't even realize it.

The simple fact is that holding the abdominal muscles in a constant state of contraction causes them to *weaken*. In order for any muscle to function effectively it has to completely relax between contractions. This holds true for the abdominal muscles. In free breathing they alternately swell and retract, allowing fresh nutrients to circulate through the muscles, and toxic waste products to be flushed out. This not only keeps the abdominal muscles strong, it helps the body to assimilate and eliminate—both functions that aid weight loss. Relaxing your abdomen doesn't mean letting it hang out in a completely flaccid state; it means letting your belly move so that you experience both the relaxation and tonus phase of the breath cycle.

Holding the Belly in Will Prevent Back Pain

If you've suffered from back pain at any time you may have been told to keep your abdomen pressed back toward the spine *all the time* in an effort to stabilize your spine. It is true that strong abdominal muscles aid the spinal muscles in supporting the back and should be used especially when lifting to stabilize the spine. However, keeping the abdomen contracted all the time *increases* the tension and stiffness in the lower back muscles and if you suffer from back pain it can increase your pain levels. The diaphragm attaches along the front of the lumbar vertebrae, so any constriction in this important breathing muscle will immediately be reflected in the function of the spine. Ironically, the only way the intervertebral discs (the spongy cushions between each vertebrae) can remain thick and healthy is by imbibing fluid (much as a sponge absorbs water). This process of imbibition can happen only through movement since there is no direct blood supply to the discs after the second decade. We need movement to keep our backs healthy and what better movement than the ongoing massage of our breaths? The oscillation of the breath also provides an effective means of giving traction to the spine, creating space between the bones and thereby reducing nerve impingement, bone degeneration, and arthritic conditions. Allowing your abdomen to move when you breathe is the most effective way to keep your back healthy.

of the body, relax and wait for the vitality of the breath to emerge rather than mechanically forcing the movement.

In the beginning it is better to allow the breath to come in and out of the mouth—this will make the movement of the breath bigger and easier to perceive. Also, if you tend to control your breath, breathing in and out of your mouth will free up the breath process. Allow your jaw to hang slightly open so that you can let any sounds or sighs release on the outgoing breath. Feel free, though, to explore breathing in and out of your nose during any part of the following exercises. Start with the lower abdomen.

Abdomen (Figure 11) Your helper should now broaden the fingers of one hand and press firmly on your lower abdomen. Or you can place your own hand

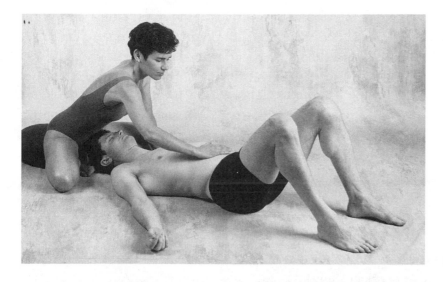

FIGURE 11

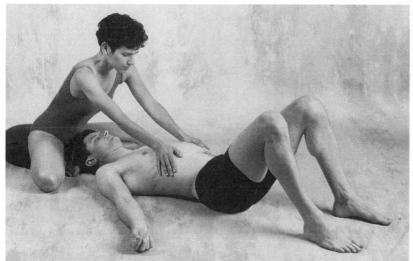

FIGURE 12

on your belly. Let your breath begin to rise in this area. Notice if this movement feels familiar or unfamiliar. Is it easy to breathe here, or does it feel like an effort? Take up to three minutes exploring how the breath moves in this part of your body. As you take the pressure of the hand away, continue to breathe in the area you have just touched. Can you breathe here without help?

Diaphragmatic Movement (Figure 12) With both hands your helper can now cup the lower rib cage with the thumbs touching the inner borders of the ribs and the fingers wrapping around the outsides of the ribs (but not the soft tissue in the depression underneath the tip of the sternum). If you are doing the movement by yourself, reverse the movement of the hands so that your thumbs wrap around the lower rib cage with the fingers facing each other. Let your breath begin to rise in this area, feeling your skin make contact with the entire surface of your own or your partner's hands. Allow the movement to be felt throughout the sides of the rib cage as well as the front. Notice if this movement feels familiar or unfamiliar. Is it easy to breathe here or does it feel like an effort? Take up to three minutes exploring how the breath moves in this part of your body. As the pressure is taken away, continue to breathe in the area you have just touched. Can you breathe here without help?

Intercostal Movement (movement of the rib cage) (Figure 13) Now have your helper move her hands onto the sides of your rib cage, just underneath the armpits. You may want to bring your arms further away from your body to make more room for your partner's hands. Your helper is going to press her hands against the sides of the rib cage. Alternately you can press your own thumbs against the upper ribs just below the armpits. Explore what it feels like to breathe into the sides of the rib cage. Is this a familiar or unfamiliar movement to you? Is it easy or does the act of breathing here take great concentration? Can you feel

FIGURE 13

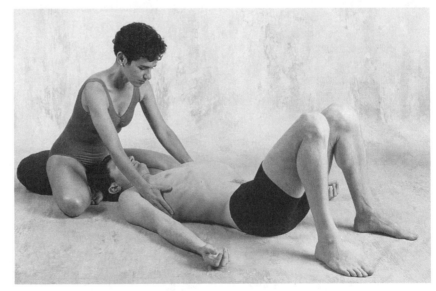

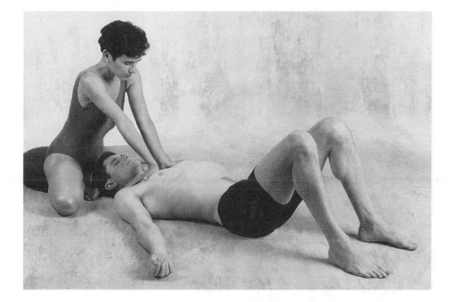

FIGURE 14

the spaces between your ribs expanding on the inhalation and retracting on the exhalation? Take up to 3 minutes exploring how the breath moves in this part of your body. As you take the pressure away, continue to breathe in the area you have just touched. Can you breathe here without help?

Upper Chest Movement (Figure 14) Next have the helper move her hands to the center of the upper chest, just below the collarbones either side of the sternum. Her hands should not press down toward your belly but should suggest a slight upward movement toward your throat. The helper should make sure that her fingers are not pressing on the delicate area above the collarbones or on the throat in any way. If you are doing this alone press your fingertips against the upper chest.

Let the vitality of your breath arise from this part of yourself. Does this movement feel familiar or unfamiliar? Do you find yourself struggling to breathe in this area, or is it quite easy? Take up to 3 minutes exploring how the breath moves in this part of your body. As you take the pressure away, continue to breathe in the area you have just touched. Can you breathe here without help?

Cranial Movement (Figure 15) Now your helper can put her hands around the back of your head, cupping the skull while letting it rest on the ground.

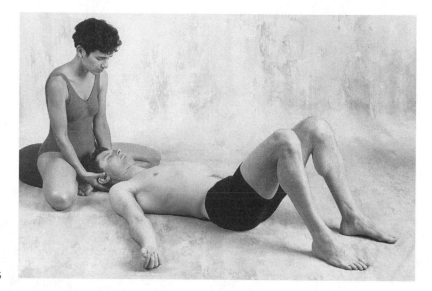

FIGURE 15

Alternatively, place your own hands around the sides of your skull in any position that is both comfortable for your hands and for your head and neck. Imagine your brain like a lightbulb—glowing bright on the inhalation and dimming on the exhalation. Feel your cranium, especially in the back of your skull, expanding and broadening as you breathe in and condensing as you breathe out. Your helper should keep her hands firm but relaxed so you can allow the full weight of your head to release into the floor. Especially notice whether you can feel the back of the skull broaden and soften with each exhalation. Take up to 3 minutes exploring how the breath moves in this part of your body. As you take the pressure away, continue to breathe in the area you have just touched. Can you breathe here without help?

Returning to the Beginning Just as you did at the beginning of this inquiry place one hand on your lower abdomen and one hand on your chest. Try to be specific in answering the following questions. Do you notice more movement underneath either hand? Has your breath pattern changed in any way? Is the movement of your breath more equally distributed between the top and bottom halves of your torso? Has the *quality* of your breath changed in any way? Can you describe the difference between when you started the inquiry and now? Do you feel different and if so how? Take a few moments to relax before rolling on your side and sitting up.

Before you move on share with your partner how you perceived your breath. Where did it feel difficult to focus awareness and expand the breath? Where were you most adept? Let your friend relate her perception of what she saw and felt. Often the two impressions differ. If you are working by yourself make notes of what you observed. Remember this is not a time to interpret or evaluate any of these observations. It is simply a time to notice. If you are in the helping role, refrain from giving psychological analysis or interpretations of your partner's breath pattern.

Characteristics of Free Breathing

Now that you have a general idea of your own breathing you may be thinking, "But what is the *best* way to breathe?" The best way to breathe is the way that supports the activity that you are doing. If you are presenting an important proposal to your boss, your breath will need to be quite different than if you are singing a lullaby to your child. Free and effective breathing does, however, have certain characteristics. Some of these are:

- **Oscillation** The whole body oscillates and moves slightly during free breathing. This movement arises effortlessly and not from suppressing movement somewhere else. The oscillation has a way of traveling sequentially through the body from the center to the periphery.

- **Diaphragmatic** The breath arises predominantly through the action of the central diaphragm rather than through the action of the more external secondary respiratory muscles, which are higher up in the body.

- **Internal Origination** The breath arises from within rather than being pulled inside mechanically by using the outer muscles of the body. Instead of breathing we are breathed.

- **Multidirectional** The breath expands in all directions, radiating out, just as a full dandelion flower radiates from its core.

- **Calm and Regular** The breath has a feeling of being and creating calm in the body and mind. Its rhythm is regular most of the time.

- **Two/Three/Pause Rhythm** During quiet respiration it's normal for your inhalation to be about 2 seconds and your exhalation to be about 3 seconds followed by a pause. More simply, you breathe out a little longer than you breathe in.

- **Flexible** Just as waves arise in endless variation in the sea, the breath arises with endless variation and adaptability. The breath changes as our thoughts, feelings, and movement change.

- **Effortless** The act of breathing is filled with a sense of ease and relaxation.

While there is no one "correct" way to breathe, there are more and less effective ways of breathing. To understand this it will be helpful to pause for a moment and look at some of the structures that support effective breathing.

III

The Anatomy of Breathing

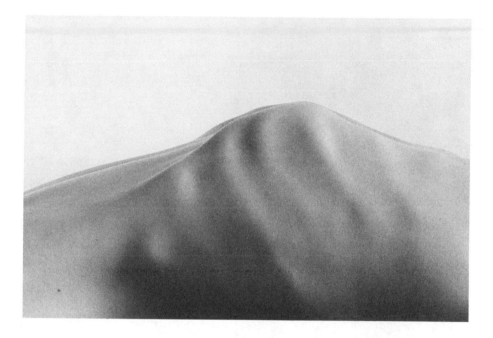

No one has form without breath. Consequently, breath and form must be accomplished together. Isn't this evident?

—MASTER GREAT NOTHING OF SUNG-SHAN,
TAOIST CANON ON BREATHING

*M*ost of us have had some education about the anatomy of our bodies, which was usually taught to us as dry, boring material that needed to be memorized like the capitals of distant states. But rarely, if ever, were we asked to *experience* our structure. You are this information! This essential perspective is unfortunately lost on our educators and so we arrive as adults, knowing vast amounts of irrelevant information, yet knowing nothing about ourselves and the body that must carry us throughout our lives. This chapter on respiration is not intended to be comprehensive or theoretical. Rather, it is intended to help you have an experienced understanding of the anatomy of your breathing. So as you read the information in this chapter pause frequently to visualize these structures in your own body. Put your fingers on your body and feel where these structures are. Don't be satisfied with being a passive receptacle for information. I think it's extremely important to allocate lavish amounts of time and energy in the service of knowing about your body and how it works. This experienced knowledge of your body is the best health insurance policy you will ever acquire.

Going Inside the Body

It is the cells that desire the breath.[1] When air enters our bodies it takes a circuitous path through the body, moving through different passages, chambers, tubes, organs, and gradually branching off into smaller and smaller tributaries until it reaches the cells. Cells need energy and they acquire it through the nutrients we eat and through a constant supply of oxygen. Oxygen rides on the back of hemoglobin in the blood until it reaches the tiny thin-walled capillaries. It is at the level of the capillaries that oxygen is given up into the tissue and exchanged for carbon dioxide. This deoxygenated blood, which looks bluish, flows back though the veins, traveling into larger and larger blood vessels until it reaches the heart, where it is once again pumped out to the lungs to receive new oxygen.

While the lungs and heart must work in synchrony with one another to circulate oxygen throughout the body, it is the respiratory muscles that actually draw the air into the body. These muscles are like any other muscles in the body—they can become chronically tight and shortened, they can weaken and have poor tone, and they can move in a distorted way if they are being asked to take over tasks they were not designed to do. While we may easily notice tension or tightness in our neck and shoulder muscles, it takes a more refined awareness to feel the condition of our respiratory muscles because they lie so deep within the body.

> Internal respiration or cellular breathing . . . establishes the integrity of each cell and its relationship to its internal fluid (sea) environment. External respiration or lung breathing . . . establishes our own personal separateness and our relationship to our external air environment.
>
> —BONNIE BAINBRIDGE COHEN, *SENSING, FEELING AND ACTION*

Primary and Secondary Respiratory Muscles

To become more sensitive to these structures it is helpful to visualize them clearly. In the human body the respiratory muscles are categorized into two groups: primary (essential for full breathing) and secondary. The primary muscles, which are lower in the torso, do the bulk of the work and are generally very large and strong as they must work over 22,000 times each day. Like the heart, which beats every minute of our life without tiring, the kingpin of breathing, the diaphragm, also toils relentlessly without fatigue. The secondary muscles, which are higher up in the body, act as auxiliary helpers and play an important role in giving us greater adaptability in our breathing. Generally they are smaller and more delicate muscles, but can act powerfully for short periods of time if called into action. They also may be active during very quiet respiration. Unlike the diaphragm, these secondary muscles tire quickly and easily. The most important

The first person is using his primary muscles to do 80 percent of the work and letting the secondary muscles help out with 20 percent effort. Notice the stability of the triangle with its base facing the ground. The second person is using his secondary muscles to do almost all the work and leaves the primary movers to contribute a paltry 20 percent of the effort. Notice the instability of the triangle with its tip facing down. When you breathe with the lower muscles you *are* more stable.[2] When you focus your attention and breathing action in the lower body you also have the subjective feeling of being more "grounded." Try both ways of breathing and see which one makes you feel grounded and which one makes you feel as if you have your head in the clouds. Also observe how the increased energy in the upper body literally keeps you "in your head" and that as you focus your attention on the lower body you become more in touch with your "gut feelings." This is how we embody the expression being "out of touch with our feelings" or "following our gut instinct." Whenever you feel confused about your feelings, bring your breathing down into the lower body, low and slow, and see what happens.

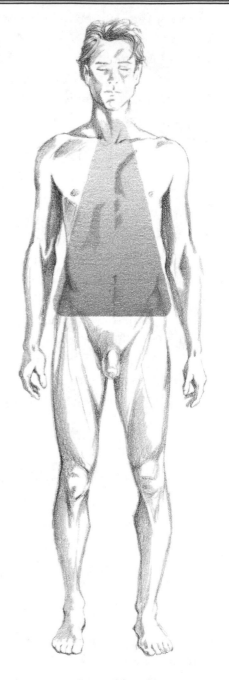

8. *Optimal breathing*

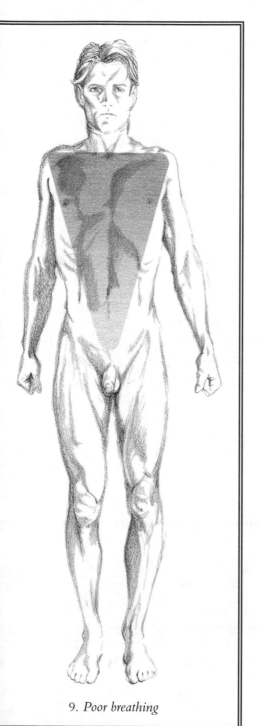

9. *Poor breathing*

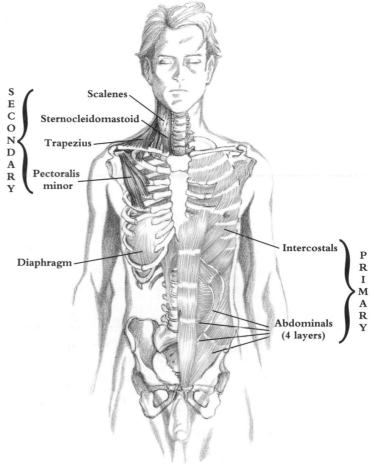

S
E
C
O
N
D
A
R
Y

Scalenes

Sternocleidomastoid

Trapezius

Pectoralis
minor

Diaphragm

Intercostals

P
R
I
M
A
R
Y

Abdominals
(4 layers)

10. *Primary and secondary respiratory muscles*

thing to remember about these two muscle groups is that their roles should *never be reversed.* The secondary breathing muscles should never be asked to take on the role of prime movers.

The principle muscle that is responsible for 75 percent of all respiratory effort is the *diaphragm. (*A diaphragm is any muscular, membranous, or ligamentous wall that separates two spaces.) It is assisted by the other primary muscles— the *intercostals* between the ribs and the *abdominal* muscles that girdle the front of the belly. The secondary respiratory muscles are the thin *scalenus* in the front of the neck, which attach to the upper-most ribs; the *pectoralis* in the chest, which body builders love to develop; the *sternocleidomastoid* running from the mastoid process from just behind the ear to the top of the sternum and clavicle; and the *upper trapezius,* which run from the base of the skull to the top of the shoulder blades, which most of us know well as tightropes of tension that gird the upper body.

The Diaphragm

Because the diaphragm is so important we will focus most of our attention on where it is, what it does, and how it moves.

The diaphragm is a huge double-domed shaped muscle that sits in the chest like a parachute. If you were to cut the body in half and remove the abdominal organs, you would see a glistening bowl-like structure with radiating fibers from the center of the dome to the outer edges of the body. A central tendon marks the top of the dome, which is whitish in color and slightly flattened to make room for the heart, which sits above. Just like the panels of a parachute, the fibers of the diaphragm radiate out from this central tendon. They attach in the front to the inner surface of the xiphoid process (the little bone at the end of your breastbone); throughout the sides on the inner surfaces of the cartilage of the seventh through twelfth ribs; and all the way down the front of the spine by way of long tendinous *crura,* which attach to the first to the fourth lumbar vertebrae. The crura act like anchors for the diaphragm much in the same way that a handle secures an umbrella. The crura muscles in particular give us some clues as to why breathing can move structures as far down as the tailbone. Take a moment to visualize where the diaphragm is in your body.

The organs above the diaphragm need to be connected and in communication with the organs below the diaphragm, so there are openings to allow for the

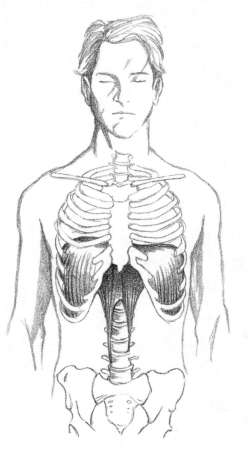

11. *The diaphragm*

passage of blood vessels, nerves, and the esophagus. The Native American Indians saw the diaphragm as the horizon between heaven and earth, and in many ways this analogy is fitting. Our heart and brain reside above the diaphragm and our guts and sex organs sit below. The heart and lungs lie just above the diaphragm and are responsible for your circulation and respiration. The stomach, pancreas, gallbladder, and small intestine lie just below the diaphragm (the stomach being on the left side) and are responsible for digestion and assimilation, while the large intestine and sigmoid colon take care of reabsorption and elimination. The liver is just below the diaphragm on the right and acts as the chief processing and recycling plant of the body, breaking down poisons and storing important nutrients. The spleen, which lies on the left side next to the stomach and directly below the diaphragm, has an immune function since it contains cells that destroy harmful bacteria. It also recycles worn out blood cells as well as pro-

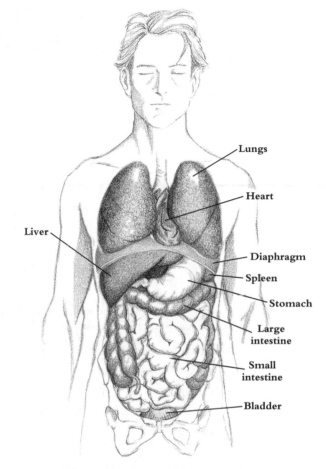

12. *The organs above and below the diaphragm*

ducing new ones. In the back of the body near where the diaphragm inserts, the kidneys are filtering and regulating the concentration of water and solutes in the blood as well as excreting wastes in the form of urine. Further down are the reproductive organs—the testes and prostate glands or the ovaries and uterus.

When the diaphragm moves in the luxurious expansions that mark full breathing, all these organs are massaged, rolled, churned, and bathed in new blood, fluids, and oxygen. The organs get squeezed and released like sponges. Breathing stimulates all of the body to work better and this is why it has such a profound effect on our sense of well being. Subjectively this free movement in the inner body also allows for communication between the rationale/thinking aspect of ourselves and our instinctual/animal nature. Take a moment as you sit to feel the way the organs in your body migrate with the ebb and flow of the breath current. Looking at the illustration place your hands on the surface markings of each organ and feel the way the organ moves as you breathe.

How the Diaphragm Moves

The position and shape of the diaphragm depends on the phase of respiration, the position of the body and also the degree of fullness in the soft organs. Because of its deep central position, its movements are not directly visible but must be inferred by the movements on the surface of the body.

When we inhale the diaphragm lowers, displacing the soft contents of the belly and thereby creating a larger space in the chest. As this space is created, the pressure in the atmosphere exceeds the pressure in the chest and air flows inside to balance these pressures. To exhale completely, the diaphragm must relax and billow back up into the chest, compressing the air in the chest and allowing the air to be expired. The diaphragm not only moves up and down, it also broadens and fans outwards. For air to move in and out freely the diaphragm must be able to expand without being restricted. As we shall see, there are many ways that we can limit these excursions. By doing so we limit not only the movement of air into and out of the body, but the rhythmic massaging action which the diaphragm exerts on the organs.

The Pelvic and Vocal Diaphragm

Traditionally, the diaphragm that separates the thoracic and abdominal cavities is the only one that was considered important for breathing. There are, however, two other diaphragms that play important roles in allowing the most central diaphragm to work effectively. These are the *pelvic diaphragm* and the *vocal diaphragm*. You might imagine the three diaphragms as domes that lie perpendicular to the vertical axis of the body.

The pelvic diaphragm that makes up the pelvic floor is best known for its function in supporting the weight of the pelvic organs and for its dynamic role in closing the rectum. The vocal diaphragm, located at the top of the trachea, is best known for its role in phonation (making sound). Both are less known for their role in facilitating full body breathing.

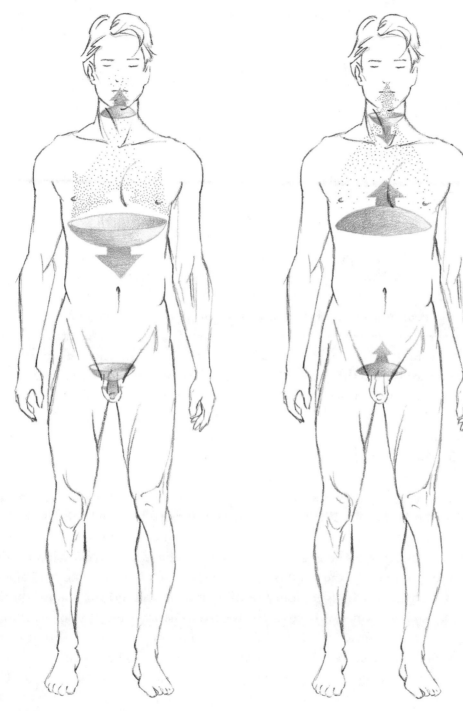

13. *The three diaphragms on inhalation*   14. *The three diaphragms on exhalation*

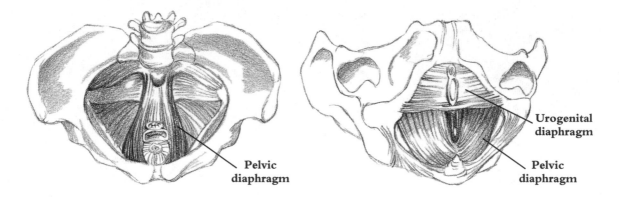

3.6 The pelvic floor

The pelvic diaphragm is like an inverted parachute that lies at the funnel-like opening at the base of the pelvis. The pelvic floor actually consists of two diaphragms—the pelvic layer and the urogenital layer. The muscles of the pelvic diaphragm run roughly from the pubic bone in the front to the tail in the back. This layer is the deeper of the two, with many of its muscle fibers running circularly around the anus and genitals. Closer to the surface, the urogenital diaphragm runs from the inside of the sitting bone on the right side to the inside of the sitting bone on the left. There are openings in both diaphragms to allow for the sexual organs, urinary tract, and anus. When we inhale, the pelvic diaphragm billows downward and broadens, and when we exhale, it retracts upward and narrows.

The vocal diaphragm is a disc-shaped structure situated in the upper part of the air passage between the trachea and the base of the tongue. When we breathe, the vocal folds draw apart, and when we make sound the vocal folds come together. Long, lax cords produce a low-pitched sound, and short, tense cords give higher tones. The glottis (the little flap above the larynx that prevents food from going down the windpipe) also opens when we breathe in and closes when we breathe out. When your breathing is deep and relaxed you may have noticed that your voice is deep. You might notice after breathy love-making that your voice is fit for a Marlene Dietrich audition. Similarly, when you are very nervous and your breathing moves only in the upper chest, your voice may become high and squeaky. When people strain while exercising it is possible to hear the holding in the back of the throat as a a "hmmph" sound on the exhalation.

16. *Follow the pathway of your important breathing muscles starting with your sternum. Find the tip of your breastbone and mentally follow the path up into the dome of your diaphragm, sensing the top of the diaphragm where the heart sits. The diaphragm then descends down the front of the spine. Trace your fingers down from your waist in the back until you come to the sacrum. Continue down, find your coccyx, the tailbone, and pick up the trail again by palpating the pelvic floor muscles, from the tailbone through to the anus and genitals until you touch the pubic bone in the front. Pick up the trail again by following the rectus abdominus muscles, which attach at your pubic bone and insert at your xiphoid process (the tip of your sternum). Feel the other abdominal muscles to the left and right of center and finish by feeling along the sides of your rib cage where the intercostal muscles are and the costal portion of the diaphragm inserts. Follow the diaphragm back to the top of the dome where the heart sits. Well done! You've completed the breathing circuit.*

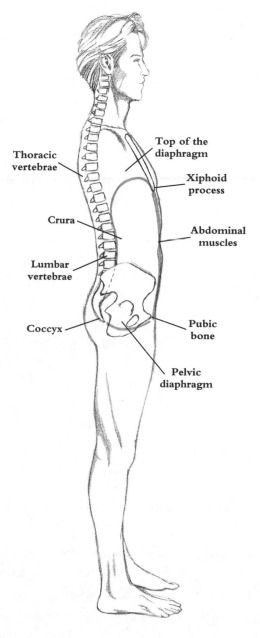

The Anatomy of Breath Holding

Remember that the primary diaphragm must be able to broaden and move freely up and down in order for you to breathe effectively. Any pressure exerted from above or below the diaphragm would limit its movement. During relaxed breathing the diaphragm descends during inhalation, causing the belly to widen and expand outward. Both the pelvic and vocal diaphragms respond to this movement by opening outwards (vocal cords and glottis open out, and pelvic muscles release and spread). (See Illustration 13.) When we exhale, the diaphragm ascends back up into the chest, drawing the abdomen inward and slightly upward. The pelvic diaphragm responds by drawing in and up and the vocal diaphragm by closure of the glottis. (See Illustration 14.) Imagine the diaphragms like circular doors that blow open or shut depending on which way the wind is blowing. The movement of any one diaphragm affects all the others.

When the abdomen is chronically tightened and pulled inward and upward, as is so common in Westerners, the pelvic diaphragm is also held in a state of chronic contraction. The anal sphincter muscles become tight and are pulled in and up (giving new meaning to the expression "a tight ass"); the urogenital and perineal muscles contract and move upward. When the pelvic diaphragm is upwardly inverted *all the time* a curious phenomenon takes place. Since the primary diaphragm is unable to complete its downward excursions, the secondary respiratory muscles are required to take over the work of the diaphragm. Using these muscles to breathe deeply is rather like using a fork to dig a hole. It's very tiring and very ineffective. Because the primary diaphragm cannot move freely downward our ability to inhale is radically reduced. When we can't inhale completely we tend to exhale quickly (and thus not completely) in order to grab for another inhalation in the hopes of getting more air. A cycle is set up whereby the harder we try to breathe the less air we get.

Situated as it is at the top of the throat, the vocal diaphragm has a more subtle action upon the thoracic diaphragm. Holding tension in the throat and vocal diaphragm indirectly affects the ability of the central diaphragm to move freely up and down. Imagine now, all three diaphragms hovering over one another. If we close and press downwards with the vocal diaphragm the central diaphragm reacts by reducing its excursions both up and down, and if we pull upward with the pelvic diaphragm the central diaphragm can't descend completely so that we can't breathe in fully.

All these strategies force us to breathe with irrelevant muscles rather than the diaphragm.

How Do You Know When You Are Breathing Improperly?

We'll look at this question in detail in chapter 4, but in general, you'll feel a great deal of tension in your upper body. You'll tend to accumulate tension in your neck and shoulders and between your shoulder blades in your upper back. You may even feel tension in your jaw, facial muscles, and around your eyes, possibly in the form of a headache. These are but a few of the symptoms of poor breathing, which can be as extreme as the sensation of having a heart attack.[3] No passive massage or physical therapy will remedy this chronic tension for it will be recapitulated the moment you continue breathing poorly.

Breathing and the Heart

If neck and shoulder tension were the only by-products of poor breathing we might not have much to be concerned about. It turns out, however, that poor breathing can cost us our lives! There have been a number of significant studies showing a correlation between upper chest breathing and heart disease. In one stunning report, patients who had already experienced a heart attack were taught how to breathe diaphragmatically and to generalize this behavior into everyday activities. In doing so they significantly reduced their chances of having a second heart attack.[4] Another study showed that all 153 patients of a coronary unit breathed predominantly in their chests.[5] Similarly, essential hypertension (high blood pressure of unknown cause) has been shown to respond favorably to a regimen of diaphragmatic breathing.[6] The anatomy of the heart in relationship to the diaphragm gives us some clues as to why full diaphragmatic breathing would have such a positive effect on us.

The heart lies right on top of the central tendinous portion of the diaphragm and, curiously enough, is attached to the diaphragm by fascia. Each time we breathe the heart is massaged. As Dr. Andrew Thomas postulates in a recent extract in the *Journal of the International Association of Yoga Therapists,* The fact that the heart is fascially bound to the diaphragm directly, and indirectly to the sternum and lower neck joints, would seem to be a device intended to ensure manipulation by diaphragmatic action. Were this not so, it would have been a simple matter to detach the heart from the diaphragm and anchor it to a rigid structure such as the sternum. The fascial connection is so widespread that it is clear that any diaphragmatic movement will cause heart migration and, it is reasonable to assume, cause changes in shape—a sort of *built in heart massage* [author's emphasis] . . . because the Vena Cava (the blood vessel that returns blood to the heart) pierces the diaphragm, the action described above causes the Vena Cava to be increased in size momentarily, which in turn reduces pipe blood pressure and allows an acceleration of blood flow back to the heart. The fully and correctly operating diaphragm is thus a second heart.[7]

Considering how well designed we are as breathing animals one might think that the likelihood of breathing badly is about the same as catching a rare tropi-

> God formed man from the
> dust of the ground, and
> breathed into his nostrils the
> breath of life, and the man
> became a living being.
>
> —GENESIS 2:7

cal disease. Would that this were so. Even the most casual observer will discover that chest breathing is ubiquitous throughout the industrialized West. When we restrict the normal downward movement of the diaphragm through holding patterns or through hyperventilation, these distortions affect our heart function, but we cannot underestimate the possible consequences of poor breathing on all other body systems.

There are a plethora of health problems and diseases in which poor breathing habits are causative or contribute to the continuation of the problem. Treating the *symptoms* of poor breathing rather than the underlying cause is rather like giving someone with a kidney infection topical antibiotic ointment. And as medical practices have become more technologically based, many illnesses that require breath retraining are now treated expediently with drugs, which, of course, have their own side effects—some fatal. Today, the medical community too often prescribes tranquilizers, anti-ulcer medications, and sleeping remedies for conditions that would respond favorably to breath retraining.

As it turns out, we have reasons for such distorted breathing habits—reasons we will look at in Part Two. For now, take a moment to do the following simple inquiry so you can feel for yourself what a profound effect these diaphragms have on one another, in either allowing or restricting full breathing.

～ INQUIRY ～

The Dance of the Diaphragms

You'll Need (5 minutes)

A chair

Purpose

The purpose of this inquiry is to feel the way the three diaphragms affect one another. This will help you to recognize how breathing can become restricted and how you can correct your own breath holding patterns.

Here's How

Sit on the edge of a hard chair with your feet firmly on the ground and placed slightly wider than your hips. Take a moment to settle yourself and to check in with your breathing.

Because the diaphragm lies so deep within the body, it is not possible to palpate it easily. But you can feel the inferred movements of the diaphragm by placing your hands close to the insertion points of the muscle. As the diaphragm moves up and down, you'll be able to feel the way it is moving the internal organs and the surface muscles if you place your hand on the upper portion of the belly, just below the tip of the breastbone. This is where the diaphragm attaches to the xiphoid process. Feel the way the abdominal organs spread and broaden outward and downward as you inhale.

Now bring your awareness into the pelvic floor. Sense into the genitals, the perineum, and the anus and feel how these open and spread slightly on the inhalation and close and retract ever so slightly on each outgoing breath. Notice the change of pressure of these parts against the chair. Notice how the more you relax the belly and the pelvic diaphragm, the more the thoracic diaphragm can move up and down.

Now contract your abdomen and lift in and up. Strongly close and lift up through your anal sphincter muscles, and contract and lift through the urogenital sphincter muscles and the perineum. Exaggerate the pulling up of the abdomen as well as the lift of the pelvic floor. As you hold these muscles in, notice how the breath is moving beneath your hands. Feel how the shape of the diaphragm has changed as you inhale. Can you feel how the diaphragm is unable to descend completely? Sense the way that the secondary respiratory muscles in the upper back, chest, neck and shoulders are tensing as they take over the work of the diaphragm? How do you feel when you breathe like this?

Gradually release the contraction. Allow the abdomen to be full and soft again. Notice how the central diaphragm immediately responds to the release of the pelvic floor. You might try this exercise in a standing position as most people exaggerate this holding pattern even more when they are upright.

Now tighten the vocal diaphragm as you would if you were trying to hold your feelings in. Feel how the movements in the central diaphragm have changed. Did you feel how the diaphragm contracted causing both the upward and downward excursions to become smaller? Now release the vocal diaphragm and observe how the movement changes under your hand.

Take a few moments to feel your breathing with both the pelvic and vocal diaphragms relaxed. Sense the ease with which the diaphragm moves without any effort on your part. Were either of the breath holding patterns familiar to you?

The Nose

Now that you have become familiar with your diaphragms we will investigate two other very important breathing structures—your nose and your lungs. These two structures define the entryway and chambers where air enters and leaves. Examining these two structures helps us to understand why certain types of breathing are more effective than others.

We don't usually appreciate the nose until it becomes blocked. We all know how awful it feels to wake up after a night spent propped up on pillows swallowing for air like a goldfish. This unsung heroine of our anatomy does more for us than sniff out pleasant and unpleasant aromas; the nose prepares the air before it enters the delicate lung tissue so that it is at just the right temperature and humidity. Air drawn into the nose is separated into right and left caverns, and is swirled through nasal hair and along passageways lined with a light blanket of mucous that serves to catch any dust, bacteria, or other tiny particles. The air then enters a three-storied chamber. The brain, eyes, and optic nerves are just above the top chamber, the nasal cavity occupies the middle chamber, and the bottom chamber is just above the roof of the mouth. These chambers are called *turbinates* and the aerodynamics of their curved walls causes the air to swirl round and round, passing over a much greater surface area than it would otherwise. While the air is doing the Viennese Waltz in your turbinates it is picking up moisture so that it will be at just the right humidity before entering the lungs. Up to two quarts of water are supplied by the turbinates each day.[8] By the time the air has passed through these chambers it has also reached body temperature.

We also know that air alternately enters the nose through the left and right nostrils during the course of the day. Blood shifts from one nostril to the other every ninety minutes or so, causing one nostril to open and the other to become more congested. Scientific studies show that when the left nostril is open the right hemisphere of the brain is more dominant, activating the more creative, feeling side of the mind. When the right nostril is open the left hemisphere of the brain is dominant, facilitating more analytical, rational, and intellectual mind activity. Yogis observed this phenomenon thousands of years ago and developed a sophisticated practice called "alternate nostril breathing," or *nadi shodhanam,* in which they deliberately changed the flow of air through the nostrils to balance their psychophysiology. They believed that when the right nostril was open the *surya,* or sun/heating element, was dominant and that when the left nostril was open the *chandra,* or moon/cooling element, was dominant. By opening and closing the nostrils in varying patterns one could adjust the physiology of the body just like regulating a hot and cold faucet to produce warm water. Although present research on the subject is controversial, many believe that right nostril dominance stimulates the arousal-producing sympathetic nervous system and left nostril dominance elicits the relaxation-producing parasympathetic system.[9] By alternating the flow of air in a regulated way yogis could have been trying to create an equilibrium in the two sides of the autonomic nervous system and a balance between excitation and relaxation.

∼ INQUIRY ∼

Determining Nostril Dominance

There are a number of ways you can determine which side of the nose you are breathing through. One effective method is to lick your index finger and place it just above the upper lip perpendicular to the nose. As I breathe out through the nose I can usually feel which side is more open. Dr. Earnest Rossi, in his fascinating book, *The Twenty Minute Break: Using the New Science of Ultradian Rhythms,* recommends another method that I have found remarkably effective. Gently close one nostril with your thumb and then give a short and sharp exhalation through the other nostril. Do the same on the other side and then see if you can distinguish which nostril emits the higher pitch. The one that has the lower pitch is more open, although you might have to do it a few times before discerning the difference. Do keep in mind that on some occasions you breathe equally through both nostrils so the pitch could be the same.

～ INQUIRY ～

Giving Your Nose a Wash

Sinus infection has been identified by the National Center for Health Statistics as the worst chronic ailment in the United States. Thirty-three million Americans suffer from sinus disease each year, with a hefty $1.5 billion a year spent on over-the-counter drugs. Because the nose is the gateway to the respiratory system it is important that these passages be kept clean and clear to prevent such problems as sinus congestion, inflammation, infection, headaches, sore throats, and damage to the lungs. For over a century, physicians used saline rinses to cleanse the nasal passages of infectious debris. Regrettably, the advent and popularization of expensive medications to treat nasal problems has superceded this procedure; an unfortunate development because it has overshadowed a simple, cheap, and quick method that can prevent problems from arising in the first place. What the physicians of our forefathers knew is now being backed by several clinical studies that support nasal irrigation in the treatment of rhinitis (inflammation of the nose) and sinusitis (inflammation of the sinuses).

Just as you use your toothbrush daily to keep your teeth and gums clean and healthy, you can irrigate your nasal passages to protect yourself from sinusitis, colds, flu, and allergies. The mild saline cleans the passages of foreign particles, keeps the mucous blanket in the nose healthy, and stimulates the tissue to become a little tougher and thus more resistant to penetration by harmful bacteria. One proponent of nasal irrigation, Dr. David Kuhns, says that nasal washing feels "like walking along a beach and breathing salt air. It's thoroughly pleasant and, afterward, you can breathe very clearly."[10] Unfortunately, Westerners find the idea of pouring water into the nose as repulsive as the idea of having an enema in a public place. I think this is because people wrongly associate a nasal wash with the unpleasant sensation of getting water up their nose in a swimming pool, with that electric buzz in the top of the head we all remember as children. That only happens if you pour water into the upper sinuses—an easily preventable mistake. After nine months of chronic sinus infections, I personally found this a very effective remedy and now make it part of my daily routine. When I travel in polluted cities, I am also amazed at how much black dust and pollution is expelled during a nasal wash, or *neti* as the yogis call it, even when the wash is done after vigorously blowing the nose. A nasal wash also feels wonderfully cleansing after being in a dusty environment. And it is very easy to do.

The nasal wash is usually done with a tiny porcelain or metal teapot called a *neti* pot. You can purchase them at India food supply stores, Ayurvedic clinics, or through mail order (see Resources for suppliers of *neti* pots). Fill the pot with lukewarm tap water and add a good pinch (about ¼ tsp.) of non-iodized salt. Using the mirror above your sink for guidance, put the spout into one nostril and tip the head slightly to one side. Do not try to assist the flow of water by inhaling through your nostrils. Just let the water flow while breathing through your mouth. If fluid flows into the back of your throat simply spit it out. The water will flow up and out the other nostril.

When there is heavy congestion it may impede the irrigating process, but repeated use will gradually loosen the blockage. Experiment with tipping your head sideways and slightly forwards until the water finds its way up and out the other nostril. It shouldn't go all the way into the upper chambers of your turbinates or it will cause an unpleasant tingling sensation in the top of the head. If this happens you are tipping your head too far backward. It may take a little experimentation to get just the right angle so don't worry if you don't get it just right the first time. After you have emptied the *neti* pot, pause and blow out freely through both nostrils into the sink. Don't close both nostrils or you may blow the water back into the Eustachian tubes of your ear. Make a new batch of water and salt and do the other side, finishing by blowing out any remaining water into the sink. If necessary blow very gently into a tissue without pinching the nostrils closed to expel the last drops of water.

Once you get the knack, *neti* only takes a minute to do, and will leave your nose open, your breathing free, and your mind feeling clear and alert.

You can do a *neti* wash before trying some of the more advanced breathing exercises in later chapters. It is particularly effective to do a wash before practicing alternate nostril breathing in chapter 6.

Your Lungs and Your Rib Cage

Surrounded by the protective armoring of the ribs and breastbone your lungs live inside your chest, peaking about an inch or so over the tops of your collarbones in the front and extending as far down as your tenth thoracic vertebrae in the back. If you stand and put your hands on the back about 4 inches above your

The rock painters of the ancient caves of southern France were believed to have mixed pigments in their mouth with saliva and using rapid-fire exhalations through pursed lips, they propelled the paint onto the rocks with their breath. The artist literally breathed life into the image, projecting himself into the animal or creature and thus becoming lizard, bird, or mammal.

waist, you will be feeling the base of the lungs. The greatest diffusion of oxygen and carbon dioxide takes place in the lower lungs because of the higher density of blood capillaries surrounding the microscopic "air sacks" called *alveoli*. Since the blood capillaries are more generously distributed in the lower lungs, upper chest breathing results in a less efficient oxygen exchange than deep diaphragmatic breathing.

The rib cage attaches to the breastbone in the front and to the spine in the back. There are movable joints between the ribs and the vertebral column in the back, and between the ribs and the sternum in the front. Each rib consists of a bony and cartilaginous part. The rib cage looks rather like a magical bird cage with all its wonderfully curved bones and movable joints. For some people the word "cage" conjures up images of imprisonment or restriction. If this is true for you, you might imagine the ribs as "rib bracelets" as my associate Lynne Uretsky calls them, with the ability to move them as you might a hula hoop. As you breathe in the ribs lift and fan outward and upward and as you breathe out they draw inward and downward. Take a close look at the picture of the thorax and the way the ribs change position between the inspiration and expiration. Put your hands on your ribs and see if you can feel the way they change position as you breathe.

The ability of your lungs to expand completely is directly related to the flexibility of the intercostal muscles (the muscles in between the ribs) and the openness of the spinal column and rib cage. If the spine becomes rigid it will limit movement of the rib cage, and if the rib cage becomes rigid it will in turn limit the movement of the lungs. This is why there is such an emphasis in chapter 5 on opening the entire body, and not just the respiratory muscles. Because breathing is a whole body movement every part must act in synchrony with every other part to form the extraordinary movement we call breathing.

Having the flexibility to breathe into all parts of the body and to breathe in many different ways is the way the body was designed. For instance, breathing through the nose is preferable most of the time, but that does not mean that breathing through the mouth is wrong. When we want to free, charge, or

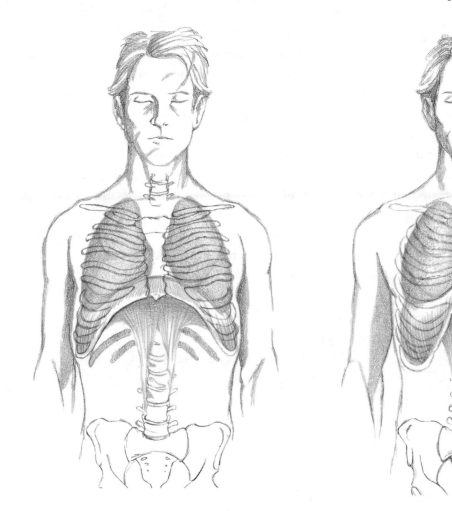

17. *The rib cage on inhalation*   18. *The rib cage on exhalation*

deepen the breathing process, breathing through the mouth can be very power-ful. It is also the kind of breathing we do when we become sexually aroused, allowing us to express ourselves with sound and to be less inhibited. Also, diaphragmatic breathing is preferable for most activities but this doesn't mean that this is the only way to breathe. It is simply an option that should be avail-able to all of us, and an option that is most underused in our culture.

Unfortunately, many of us interfere with the unique adaptability of the breathing process through particular holding patterns that lock us into one way of breathing regardless of where we are and what we are doing, regardless of how we are and who we have become. In doing so we become mechanical in the way we live and and in the way that we respond to life's inevitable changes. Habit, it has been said, is the nervous system recalling a previous experience. Like the driver who finds himself automatically driving home when he intended to visit a friend, the pathways and firing patterns of our nervous systems can drive us down the same road over and over again. This robotic way of living does not do justice to our true potential. By undoing some of these unconscious holding patterns we can begin to regain our spontaneity in the way we respond to each moment, letting each breath meet the moment with freshness and innocence. "Innocence" originally meant "without injury." By returning over and over again to the essential nature of the breath we can relinquish the fixity of the past and the imagined inevitability of the future, turning back toward the opportunity that awaits us in the next breath.

IV

Catching Your Breath

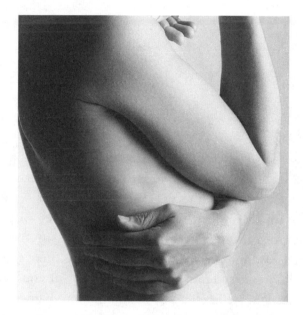

Walk slowly! Talk little! Love breath! Be thrifty with affairs! Think clearly! The body will consequently be light and the hundreds of arteries will flow and irrigate. The four limbs communicate pleasantly. The Yellow Court Canon, therefore states, "The thousand calamities disappear and the hundred illnesses are healed. One does not fear being injured by the cruel tiger or the wolf. In addition, one gets rid of old age and extends life forever.

—MASTER GREAT NOTHING OF SUNG-SHAN,
TAOIST CANON ON BREATHING

*I*t has been said that the human neuroendocrine system has changed very little since the time of cave man and cave woman thousands of years ago. Yet today we are likely to receive more stimulation in one day than our ancestors did in their entire lifetime. Whether the outer world is flying by us as we move about, or our inner mind is moving at the speed of light to cope with the phenomenal amount of information it receives, there's no doubt that the modern neuroendocrine system has its work cut out. If you live in or near any of our modern cities you are likely to be constantly bombarded by loud noises, flashing lights of all colors, and vehicles and pedestrians moving at breakneck speed and in frustratingly random patterns. Your every activity probably has been accelerated in some way, from the electric toothbrush you use in the morning to the microwave that heats your dinner in the evening. Most likely you will drive rather than walk or bicycle to work, and you will probably eat your breakfast while you do so. You will have more work than can fit into the eight hours allotted you, and at the end of the day you will travel through "rush" hour traffic, sleep to the background drone of the city, and be awakened by your "alarm" clock to start the cycle over again. And things in our ever-expanding suburbs aren't much better.

While most modern stresses are obvious to us, there are many invisible ways that modern living affects our nervous system, and thus our breathing. A recent university study has shown that simply walking on a hard surface such as concrete or asphalt causes people to unconsciously brace their bodies by tightening their abdomens, and breathing faster and higher up into their chests. It is thought that the jarring of hard surfaces increases our arousal response and thereby increases our risk of illness.[1]

There is little that has prepared our bodies to cope with this overwhelming level of stimulation and acceleration. By responding quickly and immediately to anything that resembles danger the body is doing only what it is meant to do and knows how to do for your survival. The "fight or flight" response, which I prefer to call the "fight, flight, freeze, or fake-it" response because it covers more options, is encoded in us to respond to the bear paw in the cave door, the sudden crack of a branch overhead, or the shadow of an intruder threatening our lives. The arousal response of the sympathetic nervous system was not designed, however, to be turned on every minute of the day. When we live with modern levels of stress our bodies are literally flooded with toxic stress hormones. It should not be a surprise to us that in our time heart disease is rampant, high blood pressure is epidemic, and auto-immune diseases and other ills are on the rise. While the digital clock was the emblem for the narcissistic eighties and a nation obsessed with only the present, the word *stress* and all its connotations seems to be the catch phrase for the nineties, as we propel ourselves at ever increasing speeds toward the millennium.

The responses we have to the world around us have been genetically encoded, yet we need not be slaves to either biological or cultural forces. If we are to live with some semblance of grace it will become increasingly important in our time to learn how to reorient our reactions to stress. In a sense this is an unnatural thing to ask of our nervous system given that it is receiving such a deluge of stimuli, and that is why it requires such a conscious effort.

One of the first things that happens when we respond to a stressful situation is a change in the way we breathe. Such adjustments can create as well as be the *result* of physical, emotional, or psychological stress. Disordered breathing is the absolute best indicator to us that all is not well. While it is important for us to recognize whether the stress is real or imagined, the nervous system makes no such distinctions—it only reacts. Just imagining or rehearsing a stressful situation (an activity that most of us are very good at doing) can reduce inhalation volumes. When we have been exposed to stress over a period of time, whether in the form of marathon running or divorce court proceedings, if the stress occurs for too long and with too little time in between to recover, we can forget how to relax. What was once a momentary way of breathing becomes a permanent state of being. What was once a momentary reaction is now a habit and we start to feel hyperalert regardless of circumstance, and may even continue this pattern of hyperalertness when we are asleep. How we breathe may become more a statement of what happen*ed* to us than what is happen*ing* to us right now.

Changing your response to difficulty is not as easy as you might think because for the most part you breathe unconsciously. The calibration of the nervous system's automatic pilot system can make the difference between feeling relaxed most of the time or feeling tense most of the time. You might compare the controls that govern your breathing to the thermostat controlling the warmth or coolness of your house—when the setting is off you can find yourself miserable. In your house, you can reset the thermostat to a comfortable temperature. In your body, you attempt to recalibrate the nervous system's response to stress. Ideally, you find a baseline that is maintained in non-stressful conditions and to which you quickly return after a difficult situation has passed. Most of the time your breathing is calm and regular. It may change in response to movement, activity, emotion, temperature, but you are so familiar with the baseline, that you return to it once the stress has passed. In a habituated stress response, however, there is no return to this baseline, and you continue to flood your system with toxic stress hormones. The controls that regulate breathing reset themselves to accommodate these changes in a vicious circle. Having a nervous system that is forever "crying wolf" can exhaust you to the degree that when real trouble comes you have few reserves from which to draw.

Contrary to popular belief, there is no one correct way to breathe. Dr. Erik Peper at San Francisco State University states that "any set breathing pattern is by definition pathological and does not reflect the dynamics of the system."[2] By now you know that diaphragmatic breathing is the most efficient way to breathe, but there are infinite variations to diaphragmatic breathing that could be considered normal. But before we explore strengthening these healthy breathing patterns it is crucial for you to identify your personal breath holding strategies.

There are specific and common ways that people restrict their breathing and these patterns are not difficult to recognize. When you identify your own style of breathing and free yourself of these limiting strategies you can breathe in a way that is fitting for each situation and have the flexibility to change as the situation changes rather than becoming locked into one mode of breathing.

Learning to breathe well is not an additive process in which you learn specific techniques for improving the breathing you already have. It is a process of deconstruction where you learn to identify the things you are already doing that restrict the natural emergence of the breath. Once you identify your particular holding patterns and begin to extricate yourself from their pull, your breathing will liberate itself.

In the first part of this chapter you'll focus on picking the culprit from a lineup of possible bad breathing contenders. Having done this you'll also determine if you employ self-defeating strategies in an effort to breathe more deeply. To finish the chapter there are a number of breathing inquiries that you can use to repattern your breathing with a broad brush. Later in chapters 5 and 6, you'll use a finer brush to work directly on strengthening and embedding healthy breathing strategies.

All breath holding patterns involve a partial contraction of the diaphragm. To get a general sense of how reactive your diaphragm and breathing are to stress try the following exercise.

∼ INQUIRY ∼

Contracting Your Diaphragm

Purpose

This inquiry is designed to help you feel how your diaphragm responds to stress. It will help you to identify when you are contracting and restricting the free movement of this muscle.

Here's How

You can do this inquiry sitting, standing, lying down, or in any position. Place one hand on your upper abdomen just below the base of your sternum. Relax the muscles in your body and feel the free movement of the diaphragm under your hand. Because the diaphragm lies deep in your body, you will be sensing for the inferred movement of the diaphragm, which can be felt on the surface of the body. With a quick and strong action, clench the fist of your other hand. Did you feel the diaphragm "jump" under your hand? Did you feel that it clenched just like your hand? Experiment with strongly contracting any part of your body, even your toes, and you will find that any sudden or strong contraction in your outer muscles echoes back immediately to your inner breathing muscles. When the outer muscles of body ready themselves for action, the inner muscles follow suit.

COMMON BREATH HOLDING PATTERNS

The patterns presented here are by no means comprehensive, (as each person's breathing is as unique as their fingerprint) but demonstrate some of the most common ways people interfere with their breathing. The term "breath holding" doesn't imply that you don't breathe at all but that you are restricting your breathing in some way. The patterns are presented more as caricatures of each way of breathing than as accurate statements. For the sake of clarity, I focus on the more extreme manifestation of each pattern, but they can exist in varying degrees. You need not be an emergency room candidate in a panic attack to be a hyperventilator. It's possible, if you are like me, that you often tend to breathe too fast. You need not exhibit all of the pattern for it to be true for you. When considering some of the psychological profiles of breath holders, if the cap doesn't fit, don't wear it!

Take the time before you read through each pattern to pause and check in with your own breathing. Then as you read feel whether your own breathing resembles the pattern. You can also try imitating the particular breathing pattern that is described. If it feels familiar to you, the pattern is probably quite similar to your own. It's also possible that your breathing may resemble more than one of the breath patterns outlined. At the end of each section there are general suggestions for dismantling the pattern. If you would like more specific work to correct your particular pattern, see page 201 in the Practices Guides at the end of the book.

Once you become aware of these patterns you may begin to notice the number of people around you who breathe poorly. Surprisingly, we often choose to be around people who breathe like we do for we feel comfortable in the company of others who share the same values. Have you noticed how busy people like to be around other busy people who affirm the value of busyness? The peaceful breath of a Tibetan monk tells us as much about his values as any words.

You might also find yourself attracted to someone who breathes very differently than you do for they may be pointing toward a way of being that you long for. Spending time around people who have room to breathe in their lives can be an excellent way of changing your own breathing—breathing patterns are contagious.[3]

Also, in your new-found awareness you may become a zealous observer of other breath holders. Keep it in mind that people don't usually appreciate being told about their breathing (unless they solicit this advice), and will probably find it personally offensive to be so informed. Be sensitive.

The infectious nature of good breathing became apparent to me when I began to suffer serious insomnia during one particularly traumatic year. Being a yoga teacher, I tried every breathing and relaxation technique in my repertoire but to no avail. After dinner one evening, as a close friend sat with me talking, I began to fall asleep. I noticed that his breathing was so deep and calm that just being in his presence began to soothe my highly strung nerves. I was truly amazed at the profound effect his breathing pattern had over me, especially since all other strategies had failed. On a number of particularly rocky nights when the grip of insomnia seemed inevitable, the presence of my friend's calm breathing would bring the blessing of sleep.

As you work through the patterns try not to be critical of yourself. Let your new awareness of your breathing be cause for celebration. Imagine how you might feel if you found a wallet that you were sure you had lost forever. You would be elated to recover your wealth! And so you should also be excited to reclaim the gift of your breathing.

Reverse Breathing

What it looks like

When the diaphragm descends during inhalation the downward pressure causes the abdomen to billow outwards. When you breathe in your belly should move out and when you breathe out your belly should move in. In reverse breathing your abdomen moves *in* on the inhalation and *out* on the exhalation, although you may never allow the abdomen to completely relax at any phase of the breath. The movement in the pelvic diaphragm is also reversed so that the pelvic floor *closes* on the inhalation and *opens* on the exhalation. This reversal of the natural rhythm of the breathing movement can arise from the habit of wearing restrictive clothing or tight belts and can also be the compensatory effect in advanced cases of lung diseases such as emphysema.

What it does to the body/mind

Reverse breathing causes a kind of confusion in the diaphragm and all the muscles of respiration, but it also causes a confused and disoriented state of mind. You may experience chronic tension in your upper body, especially around the back of the neck, upper shoulder, back, and jaw area. You may also suffer from indigestion, heartburn, bloating, flatulence, or a feeling of a lump in the throat. Reverse breathers often encounter great difficulty learning movement, feeling clumsy and uncoordinated because their most basic pattern of movement (breathing) is completely upside-down. Reverse breathers get particularly confused when asked to breathe in or out during a particular phase of a movement. Rather than the breath rhythm supporting movement, the breath pattern interferes with movement. They also may have no sense of *when* they are breathing in and when they are breathing out. (Imagine wearing a pair of trousers back to front and you have some idea of how a reverse breather feels!)

To test yourself

Watch the movement of your breath down the front of your body. Look at your body rather than relying on feeling your body because reverse breathers rarely can feel what they are doing. If you expand the abdomen as you breathe out you are a reverse breather. This expansion is experienced more as a collapse or drop through the abdomen rather than an opening. Also notice

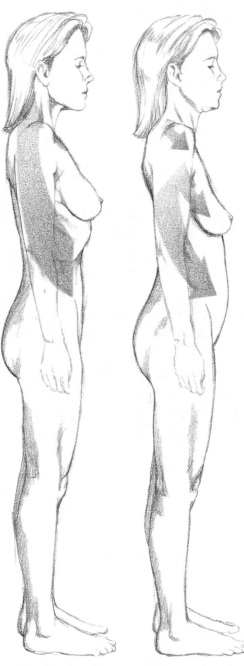

19. *Reverse breathing,*
inhalation   20. *Reverse breathing,*
exhalation

whether your breathing has a pneumatic quality to it, a kind of "heave-ho" rhythm where all the effort happens during the inhalation phase.

Dismantling the Pattern

- Consciously allow the abdomen to move *out* on your inhalation and *in* on your exhalation. You don't need to push the abdomen out or pull it in mechanically. Simply let it happen and observe how it feels to experience your breathing in this way.

- *Slow down* so you can become more aware of the reversal in your breathing pattern. Start by becoming aware of your breathing when you are sitting or standing. Then start to incorporate this awareness into the movements in chapter 5, checking that you inhale when you do movements that expand the body and exhale when the body folds or comes back to a neutral position.

Chest Breathing or Paradoxical Breathing

What it looks like

This pattern is a naturally occurring reflex that happens when you are suddenly startled or frightened. You gasp, pull the abdomen in, and breathe high into your chest. Paradoxical breathing is aptly named. The lift of the abdomen prevents the diaphragm from descending completely in order to inhale. Unable to get the air you need, you may fight even harder on the next breath to suck the air in, setting up a vicious cycle. The harder you try the less air you get.

The main pattern to look for is holding and contraction in the abdomen. This forces the breath higher up into the chest. Chest breathing is usually accompanied by the shoulders moving up and down. There may be a partial contraction of the diaphragm which allows for some abdominal and some chest breathing. Chest breathers also tend to brace the upper body, regardless if this is at all necessary for the task they are doing. Researchers have found that most people brace with their upper bodies the moment their fingers rest on a computer keyboard and that they chest breathe and increase their respiration rate while typing.[4]

Note that breathing in your chest is not necessarily pathological; the chest,

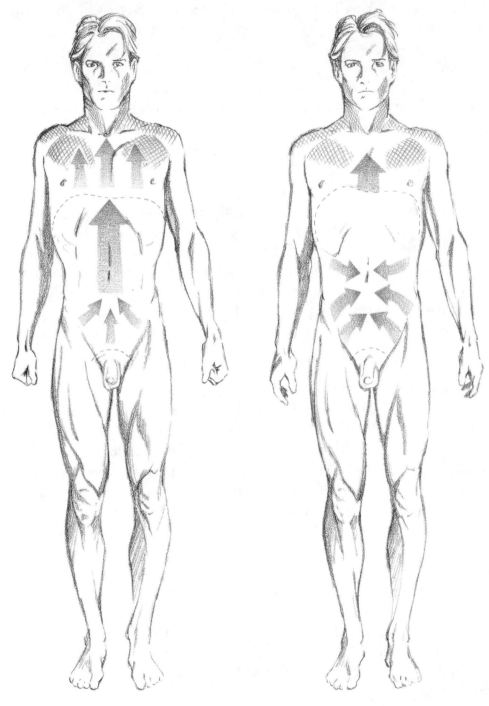

21. *Chest breathing, inhalation*   22. *Chest breathing, exhalation*

shoulders, and the entire body should expand as the breath swells from the base upwards. In full body breathing, however, one experiences this expansion as a sequential flow that creates a global sensation of expansion and retraction throughout the body. This opening is not achieved as a result of suppressing movement somewhere else. A chest breather forces the breath into the chest and will always favor breathing from this area.

What it does to the body/mind

When you chest breathe you use your secondary or accessory respiratory muscles instead of the primary muscles. Because you are relying almost entirely on these weak upper body muscles it's likely that you'll develop chronic tension in your upper back, shoulders, and neck. The accumulated tension of chest breathing is usually resistant to therapy such as massage or body work because the tension returns as soon as you resume chest breathing.

Because the abdominal muscles are chronically tightened, all the organs in the lower body suffer from a lack of circulation. One reason you may be pulling in your abdomen is that you are uncomfortable with your weight and hope that this ruse will make you appear thinner. Unfortunately, the healthy functioning of the organs of digestion, assimilation, and elimination is so seriously impaired through chest breathing that weight loss measures may be fruitless.

Men and women tend to be chest breathers for different reasons. In general, a man breathes this way as a result of a habituated stress reaction. A woman, on the other hand, may have been breathing this way since she was a young girl in an attempt to meet the ideal body image impressed upon her by peers and by the culture at large. In a recent study at Waikato University in New Zealand researchers found that children as young as nine are dieting even though few are actually overweight. Over half the children claimed to have been the subject of unkind remarks about their weight. It is not surprising that this breathing pattern often goes hand in hand with eating disorders. Those who are uncomfortable with their body weight or who suffer from eating disorders may be in a state of conflict whenever they eat because opening the stomach to nourishment means allowing the belly to relax. They may go through the motions of taking nourishment but "refuse it" at the same time with their pulled up stomachs.

Chest breathers often experience a chronic, free-floating state of anxiety. After all, this is the way we breathe during a stress reaction. Type-A personalities are often associated with this kind of breathing—the kind of person who sits on the edge of his seat and exudes "anticipation." These people never seem to have enough time to do all the tasks they have set themselves. Their chronic levels of nervousness and tension appear driven by immediate life concerns but are usually driven by deeper sources of feeling inadequate, poor self-esteem, or deep-seated fears.

As you know from the previous chapters there is a direct correlation between chest breathing and heart disease and hypertension. The most alarming thing that happens during chest breathing is that the diaphragm is prevented from descending completely, which has an immediate impact on the blood flow back to the heart. We want to breathe but we do everything in our power to prevent ourselves from breathing. Because we can't breathe in fully, we also can't breathe out fully. As a result we may resort to breathing more quickly to make up for the lack of oxygen. This sets the stage for a breath holding pattern that is even more serious—hyperventilation. Known as the "great mimic," hyperventilation has a list of symptoms longer than your arm.

As you become more aware of this pattern you may start to notice just how many people breathe this way. Chest breathing is the most common breathing disorder of our time.

To test yourself

Put one hand on your abdomen and place the other hand on your chest, on and above the sternum. Which moves more? Do you feel more movement under your top hand? Are you holding your abdomen in when you inhale? One way to gauge this is whether you feel increased tension in your shoulders when you breathe in. Do your shoulders rise with the incoming breath rather than broadening out to the sides? Movement in both chest and abdomen arising simultaneously is not usually a sign of a chest breather. Also, a sequential expansion from lower body to upper body is perfectly normal. Remember, a chest breather suppresses the breath lower down forcing it to move higher up into the body.

Dismantling the Pattern

- Release and relax your shoulders and upper back.

- Allow your abdomen to swell outwards when you breathe. Throw away (or give away) tight-fitting clothes, restrictive belts, and clothes that are too small for you.

- Take an honest look at your feelings about your body. Do you harbor unrealistic expectations about your weight, shape, or age?

- Ground yourself in the present and be aware of any tendency to hurry unnecessarily. Notice when your mind is racing into the future.

Collapsed Breathing

What it looks like

Collapsed breathers are basically chest breathers with an entirely different posture and approach. Because I personally tend to chest breathe by lifting up it wasn't clear to me that one could chest breathe downward until I observed this pattern in others. In chest breathing caused by abdominal holding the whole body moves up; in collapsed breathing the whole body moves downward. The chest is drawn downward, the shoulders hunch protectively, and the belly is projected forward and down like a dead weight. In this pattern there is too little tone in the lower body, not just in the abdominal muscles but in the abdominal organs themselves. The soft organs in the belly appear to be bloated and stagnant while the heart and lungs press listlessly down upon the belly. I frequently see this pattern in obese persons and in people suffering from depression.

In this pattern the belly remains relatively static as the upper chest and shoulders make half-hearted puffs up and down. The sound of the exhalation is often like a contained sigh. Collapsed breathers sigh and gasp frequently in an attempt to get more air.

What it does to the body/mind

In collapsed breathing there is often an intense disassociation from the body. We may be ashamed of how our body looks, or we feel so uncomfortable in our body that we exist outside its boundaries. We may have grown up believing that the body is simply an apparatus for carrying the head, and as a result disconnected ourselves

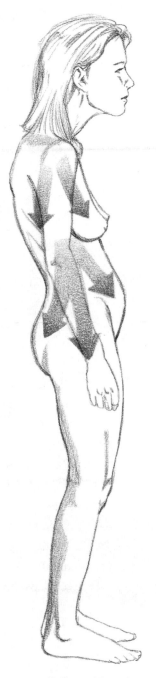

23. *Collapsed breathing*

> Melancholoke folke are commonly given to sigh, because the minde being possessed with great varietie and store of foolish apparitions doth not remember or suffer the partie to be at leisure to breathe according to the necessitie of nature.
>
> —DULAURENS, 1559

from any sensation below the neck. On the opposite end of the spectrum, collapsed breathing may be the result of harboring terrible memories of abuse and past trauma where numbing out and checking out were the primary strategies for surviving. These strategies may very well have been the best (and perhaps only) way to cope with terrible circumstances. The continuation of the pattern, however, leaves us disconnected from ourselves and disconnected from present sources of aliveness. Depression and a sense of life being a burden may be our daily wake-up call.

It is not unusual to meet people with this breathing pattern who are very lively individuals, but their aliveness seems to be from the neck up. They live in the world of ideas, and often in the world of business, where the body is seen to be of little use—some "thing" that gets exercised if there is any time left at the end of the work day. I have listened to people with this pattern speak with great animation in their faces and eyes while the body itself does not reflect or express itself either through movement or gesticulation.

To test yourself

Put one hand on your chest and one hand on your belly while you are sitting. Exaggerate collapsing the chest downwards letting the head come forward and the breastbone downwards. At the same time let the belly protrude outwards. Now press down through your feet and allow the chest to lift, opening up the space around the middle of your body. Feel the belly come alive as there is an upward lift through the central organs. Notice if the first pattern feels comfortable and familiar to you and whether the second feels strange. If you feel uncomfortable opening the abdomen and letting the chest lift, your muscles are probably very unused to carrying you in this way and it is likely that you are a collapsed breather.

Dismantling the pattern

- Unlike many of the other breath holding patterns, the solution to collapsed breathing lies more in increasing rather than decreasing the tone in the body. The focus should be on opening the center of the body. In collapsed breathing the body weight descends into the ground and is compressed by the force of gravity. By pressing into the ground with the feet, whether sitting or standing, you can create a rebounding force that lifts and elongates you through your central axis. Some of my students call this action the "Body KeBob" because it feels like a skewer straightening the body out. This internal lift also creates a psychological lift, helping us to meet the day with greater optimism and hope.

- If you found the previous exercise in opening the chest emotionally uncomfortable and you feel very disconnected or numb in your body, you may want to seek the help of a compassionate therapist. Whatever feelings lie dormant within you will most certainly surface if you begin to open your body, and for this reason it would be wise to seek guidance so you can contain the retrieval process in a way that feels safe for you.

Hyperventilation

What it looks like

Hyperventilation is not usually recognized unless in its extreme form but it can be both subtle and chronic. Dr. Robert Fried, author of *The Breath Connection,* suggests that when you are sitting quietly, your breathing rate should be about 13 breaths per minute (BPM). Men usually breathe a little slower (12–14 BPM) and women usually breathe a little faster (14–15 BPM). When we develop the habit of hyperventilating, we breathe quickly regardless of what we are doing, and our body reacts in dramatic ways to this change. This type of breathing is the natural consequence of chest breathing and has all the symptoms of that pattern, and more.

Most restrictive breathing patterns involve a partial contraction of the diaphragm. When the diaphragm cannot descend completely during inhalation it reduces the space in the chest that the lungs can expand into. With this limited lung capacity there is less oxygen with each breath. Most people will compensate for this lack of oxygen by increasing the number of breaths they take per minute.

> The so-called Yi (the mind) is the horse of the breath. When moving or stopping, they follow each other.
>
> —T'AI HSI CHING CHU,
> *THE EMBRYONIC BREATH CANON*

What it does to the body/mind

The first thing that happens when you hyperventilate is that you lose too much carbon dioxide (CO_2) from your body. While most of us know that the body needs oxygen for survival it may be a surprise to find that we also need carbon dioxide. Carbon dioxide is the crucial element in helping the body to maintain the right mixture of acid and alkaline, an essential balance for proper cell metabolism. The slightest change in the acid-alkaline balance can cause marked alterations in the rates of chemical reactions in the cells, some slowing down and others speeding up. When the body loses too much carbon dioxide the metabolism shifts from acid to alkaline.

A good example of how over-breathing can cause this shift to alkaline is when a person is climbing at high altitudes. The low oxygen content of the air stimulates her to breathe more rapidly, which then causes excess loss of carbon dioxide and the development of a mild respiratory alkalosis. It should also be noted that there are certain health conditions and diseases in which hyperventilation may be compensatory. Kidney disease and diabetes can result in metabolic acidosis and the person may unknowingly hyperventilate in an attempt to return the body's acid/base balance to normal.

Dr. Fried has researched the chain of physiological events that follow hyperventilation. He is one of a growing number of doctors who recognize hyperventilation as one of the most under–diagnosed health problems of our time. His research shows that when CO_2 decreases below normal levels (and alkalinity increases):

- The arteries in the brain constrict, reducing the blood flow and hence the delivery of oxygen to the brain tissues. (Common symptom: headache, lack of concentration)

- Hemoglobin, the molecule in your red blood cell that acts as a magnet for carrying oxygen, will tend to retain oxygen rather than giving it up to the tissues. When tissues become too alkaline the magnetism between hemoglobin and oxygen increases, thus reducing the release of oxygen into the tissue. Thus the oxygen makes its rounds riding on the back of hemoglobin but is not released into the cells where it is needed. This may perpetuate the hyperventilation pattern as the body continues to get less oxygen than it needs. (Common symptom: dizziness, feeling of breathlessness)

- The arteries in the body constrict. This results in reduced blood flow to the extremities in the body. (Common symptom: cold hands and feet)

- The increase in alkalinity causes an increase in the amount of calcium entering muscles and nerves. Excess calcium in muscles and nerves makes them hyperactive. (Common symptom: muscle tension)

- Generally low levels of carbon dioxide result in increased or over–excitability of the nervous system. The nerves may become so excitable that they automatically and repetitively fire even when they are not receiving normal stimulation to do so. (Common symptom: irritability, rushed interactions, inappropriate responses, overreaction to minor problems)[5]

Increased hemoglobin magnetism, over-excitability of the nervous system, contracted arteries . . . we might understand them with our heads, but what do they translate to in terms of how we feel? In 1978 the Journal of the American Medical Association produced a list of conditions that were thought to be related to hyperventilation. They included but were not limited to fatigue, exhaustion, heart palpitations, rapid pulse, dizziness and visual disturbances, numbness and tingling in the limbs, shortness of breath, yawning, chest pain, a feeling of a lump in the throat, stomach pain, muscle pains, cramps and stiffness, anxiety, insomnia and nightmares, impairment of concentration and memory, and not surprisingly, a feeling of "losing one's mind." If you experience a number of these symptoms you may very well be chronically hyperventilating.

Caution: There are certain health conditions and diseases in which hyperventilation may be compensatory. Conditions such as kidney disease and diabetes can result in metabolic acidosis. Hyperventilating in these conditions may be an attempt to return the body's acid-alkaline balance to normal. *If in doubt, consult a physician.*

To test yourself
Dr. Robert Fried suggests that "people who breathe normally will find they can imitate the chest movements of hyperventilators but it feels awkward." Try lift-

ing your abdomen in and up and breathing high into your chest. Does this feel familiar or unfamiliar to you?

Counting the number of breaths you take in a minute (using the normal 12–14 BPM for men and 14–15 BPM for women as a guide) will give you a rough idea of whether you hyperventilate but has limited accuracy because of the likelihood that you will try to slow your breathing down while counting. A more helpful approach is to take "glances" of your breathing throughout the day and sense if you are breathing more quickly than you really need to for the activity that you are doing. You may be surprised to discover that you are hyperventilating hours after seeing an action-packed movie or that you breathe too fast even while drifting off to sleep.

If you do not allow your exhalation to be completed before rushing for the next breath, or there is no pause at the end of your exhalation it is likely that you are a hyperventilator. Breathing through your mouth most of the time is another indication that your breathing is faster than it needs to be.

Dismantling the Pattern

- The same as for chest breathing.

- Learn to recognize when you are breathing too fast. You might want to try the "red-dot" technique. Put red dot labels in lots of prominent places at your home and office. Every time you see a dot, check whether you are breathing too fast. Are you chest breathing and/or mouth breathing too? Then focus on increasing your exhalation, breathing slow and low into your abdomen, and allowing your shoulders and chest to relax. Make sure you are breathing through your nose.

- "Deaccelerate" some of your activities. Your breathing will mirror the rate at which you do things. Each time you hear the phone ring let that be your cue to take one easy breath in and out before picking up the phone. Try parking your car a few blocks from work and walking at a relaxed pace to and from your workplace. Write a letter longhand at the end of the day instead of

> And he huffed and he puffed and he blew the house down.
>
> — *THE THREE LITTLE PIGS*

typing it, being mindful of your breathing as you write. Try driving more slowly and take the time at stoplights to breathe slowly.

• Incorporate some menial work into every day. Any task that is repetitive, and involves slow rhythmic body movement will help repace your breathing. Shoveling in the garden, sewing and knitting, kneading bread, folding laundry or ironing, and chopping vegetables are all good chores. As your breathing slows to match the rhythm of the activity you'll find your mind entering a state of tranquility.

• If you are hyperventilating because you are rushing to complete a job or task, consider these questions: Is my need to hurry real or imagined? Is this task so important that it is worth losing my peace of mind? And the clincher, Will anyone die as a result of this not getting done today? Question whether hurrying will really help you arrive at your destination or finish your task more quickly.

• The next time you catch yourself hyperventilating notice if your mind is catapulting itself into the future, planning, rehearsing, and often imagining difficulties that haven't yet happened (and may never happen). You might try reciting the short poem of Vietnamese monk and writer Thich Nhat Hanh as you breathe:

> *Breathing in, I calm body and mind.*
> *Breathing out, I smile.*
> *Dwelling in the present moment*
> *I know this is the only moment.*

• Despite popular opinion, most current authorities do not recommend breathing into a paper bag as a remedy for hyperventilation. This strategy does nothing to retrain the poor breathing pattern that underlies hyperventilation and can be dangerous in some circumstances.

Throat Holding

What it looks like

This is a more subtle form of breath restriction but can be nonetheless disruptive to full breathing. We have all felt this breathing pattern when we are over-whelmed with a wave of strong emotion in a public place and we suppress our rising feelings and brimming tears by tightening the vocal diaphragm and the muscles of the throat. Throat holding is accompanied by chronic neck, jaw, and facial muscle tension, which can be visible even to the casual observer.

What it does to the body/mind

By tightening the muscles around the throat and closing the vocal diaphragm a downward pressure is exerted through the upper torso making it difficult to allow the primary diaphragm to move either up or down. You can often hear a "hmmph" sound coming from the back of the throat when these people exercise.

Throat holders often have a great deal of tension in their voices, sounding panicked and in a hurry even when discussing the most simple matters, and their voices may be a few notes higher than normal. They may also have whispery "little girl" or "little boy" voices as they cut themselves off from the power of the sexual energy stored in the pelvis beneath the diaphragm. Some people unconsciously hold tension in their throats when they project their chins forward as a strategy for hiding a double chin.

To test yourself

Throat holding is such a subtle pattern that it is often more helpful to exaggerate the actions of throat holding, feel the effects, and note whether this is a familiar or unfamiliar feeling for you. You can also place your hand on the front of your throat and alternately contract and relax so you can feel the difference between the two states. Becoming more aware of the pattern will help you to recognize it in more casual situations.

Dismantling the Pattern

- When you notice yourself holding tension in the vocal diaphragm open your mouth and breathe out with a sigh or "ahh" sound. Relax your jaw, throat, and tongue and let your facial muscles drop as if impersonating a basset hound.

- Lower the tone of your voice by a few notes—feel your voice being propelled from deep in the belly.

- Sing! Any song will do. Practice in the shower if you are self-conscious but really let your voice fly out.

- Is there something you need to say? Is there something you are afraid to say? Take the risk to be honest and let your partner, friends, or work mates know if something is bothering you.

The last two patterns, which I will note briefly, are no less common than the others but are usually done in combination with the major patterns. They are:

Breath Grabbing

Our breath rhythm has *three* parts—the exhalation, the pause, and the inhalation. In her book *Ways to Better Breathing,* Carola Speads says that "the pause fulfills a double purpose: a resting from the effort of the inhalation and a rallying of the energy needed for the next inhalation. The pause, therefore, is not an idle period when nothing is happening; it is a vital phase in the breathing process . . . If we interfere with the length of the breathing pause, shortening it even slightly, we find ourselves feeling 'rushed' and 'pressured,' that well-known state that interferes so often with our sense of well-being and is such a generally acknowledged burden in our daily lives."[6] Breath grabbing is a term I have coined to describe the pattern when we grasp for the next breath without allowing the natural and beneficial pause.

Breath grabbers are often the kind of people who finish other peoples sentences for them. They may also be uncomfortable with allowing for pauses or silence within a conversation. We have all had the experience of jumping in on the tail end of someone else's sentence or even cutting into the last few words to start our own contribution. New Yorkers seem to be famous for this kind of fast repartee. Breath grabbers often feel that if they don't jump in or grasp for what they want, they'll miss out or be left behind.

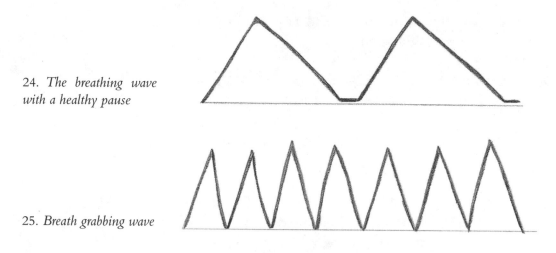

24. *The breathing wave with a healthy pause*

25. *Breath grabbing wave*

Allowing for pauses does not mean we mechanically extend the pause. You can't make a pause happen. It comes as a natural result of learning to relax into the breath and trusting that you don't need to grasp for that which will come on its own. When you allow the breath pause you are saying "I am comfortable with who I am," and just as important you are saying you are able to accept life as it comes to you. A deep, abiding sense of ease, surrender, and relaxation will arise when you allow yourself to drink in the peace of this pause.

Dismantling the Pattern

- Practice letting other people finish their sentences and allow for a pause before you speak. Observe your breathing as you listen to others.

- Is there room in your life for pauses? If not, are there ways you can restructure your time? Can you say no to new projects and responsibilities or delegate tasks to others so you have more time to smell the roses?

- Use a cue like every time you put the phone down, or every time you see your favorite color, to pause and feel the moment between your inhalation and your exhalation.

Frozen Breathing

You may have noticed that on a very cold day you brace yourself by contracting the muscles through your body. When you contract your muscles you are actually breathing very shallowly. In frozen breathing the entire outer layer of the body contracts and suppresses the rising movements of the breath, much like a snake might squeeze its unfortunate prey. Imagine your body has two layers: a softer core that is undulating and expanding with the breath: and a firmer musculoskeletal covering that acts as a container for the soft contents. When you breathe freely the inner contents and the outer container move with one another. The soft organs dilate and expand and the outer muscles and skin respond by swelling and expanding. In frozen breathing the outer container remains rigid. Very little movement is seen on the surface of the body and the body appears "frozen."

This pattern is very common in people who are very goal-oriented. "Getting there" always supersedes "being here." Such a person appears smaller than they really are, especially in the way they draw their shoulders in toward each other. These people will hold their breaths in any number of situations and often rationalize their tension by saying "As soon as this is over, *then* I'll relax!" Such a person is often so concerned with getting things right and achieving his goals, that he is willing to literally stop breathing to get there. The root of this pattern is fear—fear of not being good enough, fear of not getting there, and fear of not becoming someone.

Frozen breathing can also be a consequence of having lived in great fear for an extended period of time. The posturing here is similar to that of someone cringing or drawing away suspiciously. Children who have been physically or sexually abused, veterans suffering post-traumatic stress syndrome, and others who have lived through devastating experiences may freeze their body and breath as a way of coping with overwhelming feelings. Health practitioners and

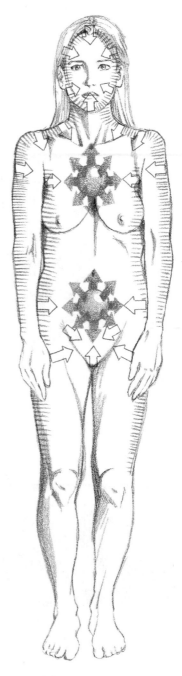

26. *The contractions and suppressions in frozen breathing*

psychotherapists working with such a person must develop his trust and confidence and work gently and gradually to "warm" the breathing process. The person must be allowed to open at his own pace so that the feelings that will inevitably arise can be integrated rather than overwhelming him as they did in the past. Cathartic methods may only result in a complete closing down.

Dismantling the Pattern

- Frozen breathers need to focus on softening and releasing the tightness in their muscles. Yoga, tai chi, dancing, and massage are excellent body practices for these people.

- Focus on allowing the breath to open from the inside of the body as you relax the outer layers. Release the shoulders and arms out to the sides and open your belly to make room for the internal expansion of your breath.

- If you feel that your breathing pattern is the result of unresolved feelings from the past, find a friend or therapist with whom you can talk.

Breathing Deeper: It's Not What You Think

We know that disordered breathing is learned behavior. Young infants and children breathe diaphragmatically until they learn to breathe only with their chests. We've been taught since an early age through the well-intentioned commands of our physical education teachers, parents, and peers to pull our shoulders back, tuck our tummy, and stand up tall! We also learned poor breathing habits by mimicking others and by being around people whose breathing process was distorted. The illustration below shows a father and his young son responding to the request to take a deep inhalation. The son has learned to copy the exaggerated lift of the chest as he lifts his shoulders as if to pick himself up off the ground.

When asked to breathe deeply most people:

- Draw the abdomen strongly in and up while thrusting the chest forward and pressing the spine forward.

- Inhale as a long "sniff." The nostrils are drawn together rather than relaxed and open.
- Move the shoulders up and down rather than laterally in and out.
- Experience breathing deeply as effortful and cease to do it once their attention has moved elsewhere.

We would do well to abandon these respiratory histrionics since they inhibit deep, full breathing. Once we relinquish these strategies the way is clear for dismantling our breath holding patterns.

Dismantling Breath Holding Patterns

Most breathing patterns are the accumulation of a lifetime's experience and they are as familiar to us as our way of walking. The nervous system has become conditioned to repeat these patterns even when the patterns are dysfunctional.

In Part Two we will look in detail at some of the unconscious forces that drive breath holding habits. For now take a moment to consider the "why" of your own breath-holding. Let this question stay in the back of your mind so that when you notice yourself in a breath holding pattern you can inquire more deeply into the root cause of your habit.

When you do notice yourself holding tension in key areas such as the throat, abdomen, pelvic floor, or shoulders, on an

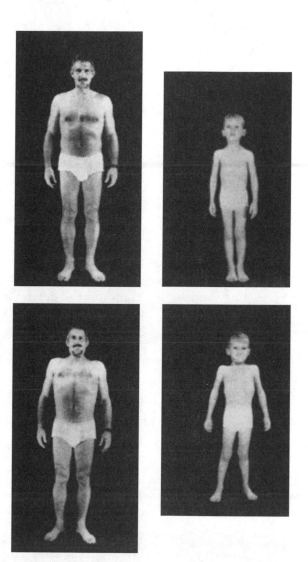

27. *"Like father like son": Breathing poorly is learned behavior. These pictures show father and son responding to the request to take a deep inhalation. Both exaggerate the lifting of the chest and spine and the propping of the body up away from the earth. Note that neither the father nor son had yet experienced the organization of their bodies by Rolfing. (Illustration from* Rolfing: The Integration of Human Structures, *by Ida P. Rolf, p. 154.)*

BREATHING AND YOUR RELATIONSHIP TO THE EARTH

Our breathing does not take place as a discrete event separate from our environment. To be human involves standing upright, in relationship to the earth and to gravity. Thus, how we physically organize ourselves in relationship to these forces determines whether we breathe well. How we breathe, and all breath holding patterns, can be understood in the context of three patterns:

> Propping
> Collapsing
> Yielding

In propping we stand on the earth like a table on a floor. We may even lift away from the earth as shown in illustration 27. This commonly results in hyperventilation and chest breathing. In the collapsing pattern, we drop into the earth without the necessary integrity through our structure to use gravity to our advantage. Here, the energy is sinking down into the earth. This results in a lethargic, labored, and shallow breathing pattern. Between these two patterns is the posture of "right" relationship—yielding. Yielding happens when we give the weight of our body to the earth but at the same time maintain enough integrity through our structure that we receive the rebound of gravity up through our bodies. You may have seen pictures of African women standing this way or know of someone who walks with an erect lightness. The dynamic pattern of yielding into the earth underlies ease and effortlessness in breathing.

Inquiry: Stand for a moment in your habitual way and observe the nature of your breathing. Then begin to tighten and lift up through your leg muscles. Feel yourself standing on the surface of the earth. As you "prop" the body notice the quality of your breathing. Then gradually let your weight collapse into the earth as if you had no bones. Notice the quality of your breathing now. Finally, try the yielding pattern, which exists in the middle of the continuum between propping and collapsing. On an exhalation feel the weight of your leg bones descending down into the earth, as if your feet could grow roots into the ground. The more you give the weight of your lower body into the earth the more gravity will effortlessly rebound through the body, creating an upward lift through the entire torso. When you yield you stand as a conducting rod between heaven and earth. Feel how you breathe when you are in this dynamic and trusting relationship to the earth. Yielding can be practiced whether standing, sitting, lying down, or in motion.

exhalation consciously relax and release these tight areas. Alternately exaggerate the tension for 7 seconds followed by releasing to clarify the difference between tension and relaxation. Removing the chains that bind the breath can be more powerful than attempting to change the breath directly by manipulating it. You are also going to the source of the breath holding patterns—your unconscious attempt to control and manipulate the way life is flowing through you. You can work with your breathing in this way at any time, in any place, and in any position, so that the dismantling process is an ongoing one throughout your day rather than something you need to schedule at a separate time.

∼ INQUIRY ∼

When Do I Hold My Breath?

Purpose

To identify the situations and activities in which you most commonly engage in breath holding. We don't usually recognize how much tension we invest in simple activities such as talking or cooking because we don't recognize the situation as terribly stressful. You may be surprised and disconcerted to discover that you hold your breath in almost every conceivable situation.

Here's How

Over the course of a week make a mental note of the situations in which you engage in breath holding. Make your observations without reproach or disap-

ENEMIES OF THE BREATH

Consider how some of these items may be restricting your ability to breathe fully. If you can't run, dance, or breathe in it don't wear it!

- **Clothes that pinch the waist** Look for clothes that have elasticized waistbands or adjustable button or tie closures that you can change as your middle expands (for instance after a large meal). Clothes that are flowing and less structured in design and fabrics that expand are breather friendly.

- **Clothes that are too small** Although buying clothes that are a size too small, or wearing clothes you have outgrown may assuage your ego, nothing looks worse than a belly struggling to free itself over a belt, a blouse gaping open, or seams stretched apart by burgeoning flesh. Men and women of all sizes look their best in clothes that fit them.

- **Belts** If you must wear a belt make sure it is not notched too tight. If the belt is too narrow it will pinch you, if it is too wide it will press into both your belly and diaphragm when you sit down. Suspenders remove the problem altogether.

- **Neck ties** Dress codes often require these uncomfortable nooses. If you must wear one, tie it loosely enough that you are not holding tension in your throat.

- **High heels** High heels throw you off your center of balance, causing the back muscles and thus your breathing muscles to tighten. If you must wear high heels, alternate shoes or minimize the impact by changing into walking shoes to and from work.

- **Bras** If it leaves red marks it's too tight.

- **Girdles & Corsets**

pointment—catching yourself holding your breath should be cause for celebration. You've made a huge leap in self-awareness. For instance, you may notice that you hold your breath when you talk to your boss. Or you hold your breath when you drive to work. Note whether the activity or situation is made easier when you breathe freely. Then try one of the following inquiries:

Moving. Choose one simple activity in which you have regularly noticed yourself holding your breath. It should be an activity where there are no time constraints or pressures, such as making your bed. Practice allowing your breath to move freely as an integral part of the activity.

Eating. Set aside one meal a day in which you do not feel any time constraints. Let yourself breathe slowly as you eat. Notice how it feels to allow your belly to release as you chew and swallow your food. Observe whether your meal is more enjoyable. If you tend to overeat or have digestive problems, did monitoring your breathing help you stop eating when you felt your stomach becoming full? How did you feel during and after the meal?

Talking. Begin to monitor your breathing during telephone conversations, noticing whether you allow yourself to pause when you need time to think, whether you allow the other person to complete her sentences before interrupting her, and whether you feel your breathing supporting your voice. Can you tell whether the person on the other end of the line is holding her breath. Can you identify her pattern? Gradually start to integrate this into more casual conversations. Your graduation exam for this exercise is to practice breathing during an argument or confrontation. How does this practice change the way you interact with others and the outcome of your interactions?

Bringing Back Your Breath

When we are in a stress mode we tend to breathe by projecting the upper chest forward, tightening our surface muscles, and reducing the length of the exhalation. All these actions follow the arousal of our sympathetic nervous system. The following inquiries work to counter these responses by replacing them with specific breathing strategies that calm the entire body. Try investigating one inquiry a week, integrating what you learn into your everyday activities.

~ INQUIRY ~

Back Breathing

You'll Need

> 2 pillows, cushions, or a folded blanket to sit on
> A partner, if you have one

Purpose

The purpose of this inquiry is to sense, feel, and expand the breath movement in the back body. Most people breathe only with the front of their body. Thrusting the breath forward into the chest often accompanies or precedes a stress response. If you tighten the muscles in the back of your body and thrust the chest forward, feel how your whole body expresses an "anticipation" or readiness for action.

When you breathe into your back, you stimulate the parasympathetic part of the autonomic nervous system. This is the part of the nervous system that is generally involved in slowing things down, promoting digestion and assimilation, rest and relaxation. Your body then thinks that all is well. Relaxing and broadening the muscles in the back of the body also releases the other half of your respiratory muscles. (A special thanks to yoga teachers Angela Farmer and Victor Van Kooten who introduced me to back breathing many years ago during one of their Greek intensives.)

Here's How

With a Partner: Once you've made yourself comfortable your helper can sit facing your back. Throughout this exploration they will be placing their hands either side of your spinal column, starting at the lowest part of the spine and gradually working their way up toward your head. As a helper, make sure that you are not pushing your partner forward. The best way that you can help your friend is to be completely present in the back of your own body. If you are thinking about other things or are distracted, your scattered attention will make it more difficult for your friend to concentrate. Also, whenever you touch your friend's back, bring your awareness to the same place in your own body and let your own breath deepen there. If you are able to breathe into a part of your body, this will be communicated through your hands, onto your partner's skin, and directly into their nervous system, without any verbal encouragement on your part. If you are holding your breath or holding a particular part of your body stiff, that too will be communicated to your friend. As you begin this inquiry, adopt the approach that you will both be actively engaged in the same pursuit—that you also will be perceiving and witnessing the breath.

Start by placing your hands, with the fingers facing downwards on your partner's sacrum. Your third finger will rest just

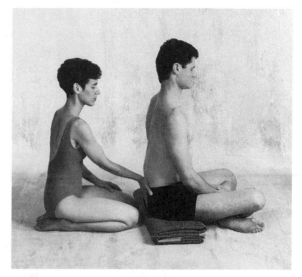

FIGURE 16

below the crack of the buttocks (Figure 16). If you want to feel as low as your coccyx, let your helper know if he have your permission to place his hand in this more intimate area.

By Yourself: Sit with your back against a wall with a pillow placed between yourself and the wall. This will give you a way to feel into your own back. Begin by sitting cross-legged, or any other position where your back is upright yet relaxed. (Or pick one of the alternate relaxation positions from chapter 2.)

Use the pressure of your back against the wall as a guide to heighten your awareness. Mentally, place your own "imaginary hand" on each segment of your back, working up from the tailbone to the back of the head, spending a minute at each level.

Both those working alone and with partners: Relax your lower abdomen and exhale through your mouth with an open jaw. This will make the movement easier to feel. First notice if you can feel any movement in your sacrum as you sit and breathe. Allow the vitality of the breath to emerge so that each area of the back begins to wake up. These are not big movements so take note of even the slightest motion. Spend a few moments sensing and feeling the breath in each area of your body. If you can't feel anything, that is useful information and make note of it. As you feel the segment you are focusing on begin to move with the breath, shift your awareness to the next level up the back.

Wait patiently in each part of your back for the breath to emerge. If you are working with a partner have your friend suggest but never insist, push, or chastise with their hands. When you have worked all the way up the neck spend some time with your helper's hands cupping the back of your head.

Notice how you feel after bringing your attention and awareness into the back of your body. Many people find that when they breathe into their back bodies their eyes become very relaxed and they have the sensation of seeing from behind their eyes. When we are in a stress mode the eyes often project forward and out, seeking information. When we come back into our center we receive rather than retrieve information from around us.

∾ INQUIRY ∾

Organ Breathing

You'll Need

A quiet place to sit

Purpose

The organ system of the body is intimately connected with the parasympathetic part of the nervous system. Terms that refer to volume, weight, slowness, feeling, and expression are the territory of the soft organs. During a fight or flight response, energy is diverted from the organ system into the musculoskeletal system to allow us to take quick action. Bringing the attention back into the organs can help return the body and breathing to a more neutral state.

In the West we tend to be more attentive to the superficial muscular layer of the body, a prejudicial awareness that leaves us largely "internally illiterate." We don't usually notice what's happening inside us until we have a serious health problem or disease. When we sense and feel the organs, our breathing automatically slows down. It also changes our perception of the breath as a mechanical action that arises from outside ourselves to an action that is arising from within us. As we become more internally literate, we start to access our own internal doctor who can warn us of trouble before it becomes serious.

The breath has to progress through the soft organs before it reaches the outer layers of the body. The movement we see on the surface of the body is only the outermost ripple of a wave that begins in the center of the body and radiates outwards through the soft organs, fluids, muscle, bone, and finally to the skin.

Here's How

Sit in a comfortable position—in a chair or on a cushion, whichever you prefer. Close your eyes and sense into the center of your body. Imagine the body as a cylindrical form with the muscles and bones as the container and the soft organs as the inner contents. You can be specific if you know the location of your organs, but this is not important. Having a general sense of the inner soft body will be enough for now.

Let yourself perceive the breath through the organs, feeling how the soft organs billow with each wave of the breath. The organs churn, slide, turn, dilate, and retract and expand with each inhalation and each exhalation. Feel how the deeper layers dilate to fill and connect to the outer layers. As you locate the breath more centrally in your body, notice if the quality of your breathing or your mind state has changed in any way.

To feel the difference between initiating your breathing from the outer versus the inner layers, shift your attention into your muscles and bones as they press against the skin. Notice how your breathing and mind state change as you move into this action system.

Shift your awareness once more into your inner body and take a few more minutes to simply sit and breathe, sensing and feeling the movement of the breath within and around the organs. When you are through with this inquiry take a moment to observe the effects of your practice. Know that at any time when you find yourself speeding up you can assist your body in returning to a more neutral place by redirecting your awareness.

～ INQUIRY ～

Lengthening the Exhalation

You'll Need

2–3 blankets or two firm pillows

Purpose

When people think about improving their breath capacity they almost always imagine that the focus should be on taking deep, impressive inhalations. Although it's counterintuitive, exhaling more fully will naturally result in a spontaneous deepening of your inhalations. This is particularly true of asthmatics who shorten their exhalation in a misguided attempt to grab for more air on the inhalation. Long, full exhalations tell the body that all is well and by consciously lengthening the exhalation we can trick ourselves into relaxing even in the most stressful situations.

Here's How

Assume the Breathing Easy position (chapter 5, p. 141). Take a few minutes to relax and settle. Then gently bring your attention to rest on your exhalation, following the exhalation all the way down into the slight pause at the end of the breath. Observe your exhalation in this way for a few minutes, letting the exhalation become like a lure to draw your mind inward. With each exhalation feel the weight of the body surrendering to the floor, allowing every muscle in the body to release its grip on the bones. Feel the eyes relax and soften and all the facial muscles release as the exhalation becomes longer and deeper. Very, very gradually, over a period of twenty breaths begin to consciously lengthen your exhalation. The total increase in the length of your exhalation may amount to only a few seconds. The idea here is to let the exhalation naturally lengthen without any strain. If at any time you feel short of breath or you find that you are grasping for the next inhalation, you are probably trying too hard. Continue until you find a comfortable rhythm where you feel relaxed and calm. You can breathe out through your mouth if this helps you. As you enter a deeper state of relaxation let go of any control of your breathing and simply watch the breathing pattern that emerges as a result of lengthening your exhalation. The whole inquiry may take anywhere from 5 to 30 minutes. Always take a few minutes to lie on your side and to sit quietly before continuing with your day.

Notice how you feel after you have done the inquiry and know that this ability to consciously relax yourself is only an exhalation away.

～ INQUIRY ～

Soft Eyes, Open Diaphragm

Purpose

Finding ways to integrate more open breathing patterns into our everyday life can be challenging. All breath holding patterns involve a partial contraction of the diaphragm. Keeping this muscle broad and released can go a long way toward maintaining free breathing. Here is a technique that you can use regardless of where you are and what you are doing. It immediately opens and broadens the diaphragm—and it might even change the way you perceive the world.

Here's How

Put one hand on your diaphragm just underneath the tip of the sternum. Take a moment to feel the inferred movement of the diaphragm underneath your fingers. Now, focus your eyes hard on a point, squinting slightly as you exclude everything from your field of vision but that one object. What happened to your diaphragm and to your breathing? Did you feel how your breathing became shallow and the diaphragm narrowed and tightened as you restricted your vision. Now, open up your peripheral vision so you sense the visual field to your sides and also slightly behind you. The moment you do this you may feel yourself take a spontaneous breath in as the diaphragm simultaneously widens. Experiment with narrowing and broadening your vision, observing how the diaphragm mimics the change in your vision.

In her book *Centered Riding,* Sally Swift uses this "soft" eyes technique to help her budding equestrians learn to relax and become more aware of the environment around them. As her students open up their breathing, the horses quite amazingly respond by calming and slowing down. In our experiment you are both the horse and the rider. I have used this technique for years in my yoga classes to help people maintain free breathing in more challenging postures. I also use it when I feel overwhelmed by the stimulation of being in a busy city street or a chaotic department store. You may find it effective in maintaining a feeling of openness when you are surrounded by the chaos of the office. The idea is not to walk around with glazed eyes; this would make you less aware of both your surroundings and your breathing. Instead, I imagine that I am looking from behind my eyes, *receiving* the images around me rather than projecting the eyes outwards and *retrieving* the images. You can also switch back and forth between peripheral focus and narrow focus when you need to concentrate your efforts. You would be surprised how open your vision can remain without sacrificing accuracy or mental focus even when doing such tasks as working on a computer. Whenever you feel yourself going into a breath holding pattern, immediately soften the eyes and open up your peripheral vision. Perhaps it will give you just the perspective you need to take the demands of the moment in stride.

Using the Techniques in Your Everyday Life

Every day we encounter situations that we find stressful, from our child screaming us awake in the morning to a near-miss collision on the way to work. These are the times to integrate some of the techniques you have learned. It's not necessary to have more than a few seconds to do successful breath work. The next time you find yourself in one of these situations, respond immediately by checking your breathing and then choose one of the options you've learned. Despite what happens to you, regardless of what life brings you, it *is* possible to maintain your equanimity. Try:

- Breathing into the back of your body
- Initiating your breath centrally through your organs
- Lengthening your exhalation
- Expanding your peripheral vision

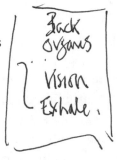

Part Two

~

Opening to the Breath

V

Room to Breathe

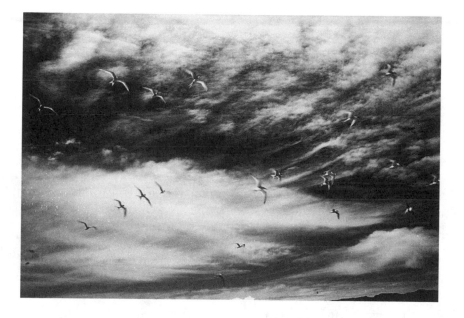

Your hand opens and closes and opens and closes.
If it were always a fist or always stretched open,
you would be paralyzed.
Your deepest presence is in every small contracting and expanding,
the two as beautifully balanced and coordinated
as bird wings.

—RUMI

*I*n this chapter we look at opening the body so that it *can* breathe and so it can receive the nourishment of the breath. Many of these movements are derived from traditional yoga postures. They are designed to stimulate your breathing by releasing and strengthening your respiratory muscles, loosening your joints, and soothing and quieting the overworked nervous system. When the opening of your breath is supported, rather than limited by your structure, breathing becomes effortless and versatile.

The entire body is designed to work in a veritable symphony of movements to insure that every part of you gets its share of life-giving oxygen. We breathe because the cells have a ravenous hunger for oxygen. For oxygen to reach our cells, the body needs to do more than simply inflate and deflate the lungs. This life-giving oxygen must be able to circulate to every cell of your body, from your brain (a particularly hearty consumer of oxygen), to internal organs such as your liver, to the outermost layer of your skin, announcing its arrival at the farthest reach of the body as a healthy pink sheen on your cheeks and in the tips of your fingers.

If your body has become stiff and tight you will have more difficulty breathing than if your body is supple and open. This tightness in the tissue and through the joints will also act as a barrier to the free flow of fluids through the body so that you do not receive the full nourishment of the breath. As the muscles and joints in your body become more mobile they allow the passage of the breath current into the lungs and throughout the body. As the intercostal muscles become long and elastic your ribs will be able to move better and thus your lungs will be able to fill with more air. As your hips become more flexible your pelvis will be able to move more freely, which will then allow the current of the breath to travel up the spine. As the spinal column becomes more flexible, the entire torso becomes a welcoming vessel for the breath. As hard and rigid muscles soften and release, the breath can move through the tissue like a fish swimming through water.

Sedentary jobs and lack of daily exercise take a big toll as stiffness and poor circulation make our bodies ready receptacles for stress and anxiety. But the way that we think and how we feel also has an incalculable effect on the tension we may harbor within. When we find ourselves constantly worrying or stuck in an eddy of repeating fears, insecurities, doubts, and intransigent beliefs about ourselves and others, these thoughts serve to build and maintain chronic body tensions. We call it tension in our body, but in reality, much of it is the recapitulation of thoughts singing their message of mayhem throughout our cells. Muscles tighten, joints stiffen, our organs don't work as well, and circulation slows as the body is flooded with the toxic chemicals that are the delegates of the stress response. All of these changes create obstacles to the free movement of breath in the body.

During the previous chapters you may have noticed specific strategies that inhibit or restrict your breath. You may have observed that you tighten the abdominal muscles most of the time or that you hold tension through the anal sphincter muscles. Perhaps you feel an overall sense of tension in your body, as if anticipating bad news at any moment, or your slouched posture makes breathing an impossibility. Keep these personal patterns in mind when you are exploring the exercises in this chapter. As you start to relax and release these chronically held areas you'll find a different breathing pattern emerging. You will also notice yourself thinking and feeling differently.

Getting Started

Instead of trying to learn all these movements in one session, divide this chapter into manageable increments, doing a few new movements each day, or even a few each week. When you have become familiar with these exercises and have a feeling for which ones have the strongest effect, feel free to creatively put together your own sequences, picking a few movements from each section. Or you can refer to the Practice Guides at the end of chapter 6 for specific routines you can follow. You'll find both general sequences for those of you in good health, and more specific sequences for working with problems such as insomnia or asthma. If you do another kind of movement practice or exercise such as tai chi, running, circuits at the gym, or you practice sitting meditation, try incorporating some of these movements into your routine. If your work or home schedule is so tight you have few spare blocks of time to devote to a formal practice, consider doing a little here and a little there throughout the day. A shoulder stretch in the shower, a diaphragm stretch over your chair during a coffee break, or a few reclining leg stretches once the TV has been shut off for the night can make a huge difference in how you feel at the end of the day.

> The softest of stuff in the world
> Penetrates quickly the hardest,
> Insubstantial, it enters
> Where no room is.
>
> —LAO TSU

If you have not moved for a long time the body can become like clay that has been left out to dry and harden. In the beginning you may feel frustrated by your body's refusal to immediately comply with your demands. It is easy to then see the body as the enemy or to feel that it has somehow betrayed you. When this happens you may resort to force by aggressively stretching your body too far, too fast. If this happens, try to remind yourself of how many times you have let your body down by ignoring its need for exercise or relaxation. Develop this compassion and your body will reward you. Gently moistening and kneading clay brings back its pliancy; in the same way the body will respond to the gentle kneading oscillations of the breath and the gradual warming and loosening of hardened muscles and tight joints. By trusting the process and measuring your success by the improvement in how you feel rather than how far you are able to go into each movement, you can enjoy the process from the very beginning. Instead of focusing on the effort, open into the pleasure, be patient, and take each movement one breath at a time.

PRELIMINARIES

BodyBreath Synchrony

In all of the movements and exercises the first and most important principle to remember is to allow the natural oscillation of the breath to be reflected in your body. Most commonly when people do exercises they breathe *underneath* the

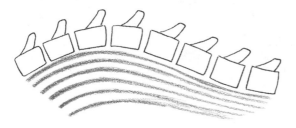 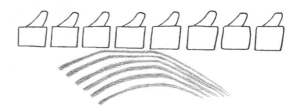

28. This represents the correct oscillation movement   *29. This represents the incorrect movement*

movement so that the outer body does not reflect the way the breath rises and falls. Illustration 29 displays what it looks like when the wave of the breath rises but the bones, muscle, and skin do not move in response. Illustration 28 shows the wave of the breath rising and the outer body moving in synchrony. In all the exercises imagine that your body is like driftwood and let it move with the ebb and flow of the breath.

The second principle is to allow the *retractive* phase of the breath to be reflected in your movement, especially when performing stretches. If you listen to the movement of your breath you will notice that there are moments when you are lifted slightly out of a stretch and moments when the breath takes you more deeply into a stretch. Most people resist the retractive or lifting phase, forcing the body to remain static, and thereby increasing the tension in the muscles. This retractive phase is just as beneficial to your body as the deepening phase. It also affords you a moment where the pulling sensation is slightly diminished, allowing you to make your stretch easier and longer. A simple way to feel this is to let your head drop down so that your chin touches your chest. Next, open your mouth and breathe in and out. Relax the back of your neck and soon you will notice that the breath is alternately lifting and lowering the head and neck. You can also try this hanging forward over your legs as in Illustration 30. This is just the kind of movement you should allow in all the exercises that follow.

When Should I Breathe In and Out?

Most texts on movement and yoga will designate a specific breath phase for each part of an exercise indicating when to breathe in and when to breathe out. One can become adept at directing the breath with the mind, but there is a greater

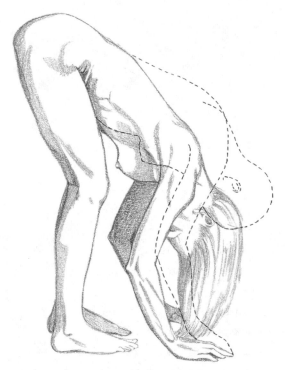

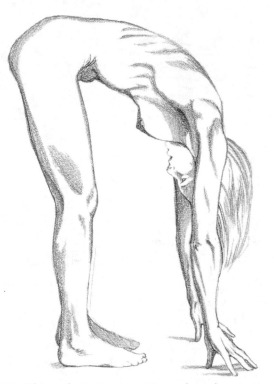

30. *This shows how to stretch allowing the breath to create retraction*

31. *This is the incorrect position, where there is no retractive phase and the body is only pulled forward*

freedom to be found in learning to allow the intelligence of the breath to emerge naturally. When you explore the movements ask:

• What is the breath asking my body to do now? What is my body asking my breath to do? Does my body want to open on the inhalation, the exhalation, or the pause in between? Generally opening, expanding, and vertical movements elicit the inhalation and closing, retracting, and horizontal movements elicit the exhalation. Go beyond rules and explore for yourself!

When I do suggest appropriate times to breathe, take these as guides rather than rules. In all the movements adjust your position to find the place where your breathing is the most open. Allow the rate and depth of your breathing to change in response to the demands of different movements rather than designating one breath for one movement and so on. Finally, never put yourself in a position in which you cannot breathe. This is good advice here and in all life situations. You can be sure that if you cannot breathe, your position is incorrect.

Find the place where the stretches are deep enough to have captured the attention of your mind but not so intense that you disassociate from your experience and enter a stressful breath holding pattern. Although it is preferable not to reach this stage, you know that you have pushed your position too far if the sensation is so intense that you cannot hold it for one breath cycle. Give yourself enough breathing space so you can open into the pleasure rather than the effort of each movement. That way, you will have positive associations with your breath work sessions and will be eager to return to them every day.

Equipment: Things You'll Want at Hand

- A chair
- 1–3 firm blankets (cotton or wool is best)
- A few pillows or cushions of different sizes
- A bath towel
- A tie (a belt, bathrobe, or necktie will do)
- A dark cloth to cover the eyes or an eye bag: Eye bags are small rice-filled bags that cover the eyes and press gently against the eye muscles to help you to relax (see Resources for suppliers or how to make an eye bag)

Optional

- A "breathing bolster." This is a cushion made especially to put underneath your spine in a reclining position. A bolster can save you time and energy in folding blankets (see Resources for suppliers).

- A *round* "yoga bolster": This is a larger, round bolster that can be used to support the body in many of the restorative positions. You can improvise with blankets or firm cushions. The convenience of a bolster will make it more likely, however, that you will sustain your breathing practice (see Resources).

- A sandbag or a bag of beans or rice: Sandbags are soft cotton or corduroy bags filled with about 10 pounds of sterilized sand. Their weight can be helpful for diaphragm strengthening exercises (see Resources for suppliers).

- A partner for some of the exercises.

On the Road or at Work

If you are on the road a great deal, you may think you'll need a donkey to carry all this equipment. Not true. Most, if not all of these exercises can be done at work and while on the road. With a little ingenuity you can improvise with what you have on hand. At the office a leather belt can become a tie, in a hotel a few sofa cushions can become back supports, and in an airplane the walls along the back of the plane can be perfect shoulder stretching equipment. A reclining exercise can often be done sitting in your car, and a sweatshirt or jacket can become a neck support in a pinch. I travel four to five months of the year and find that almost every household or hotel I stay in has more than enough "equipment" for me to continue my daily wellness practice. It's not difficult to do, but you do have to decide that you *want* to do it. The degree to which you believe you do not have the time, or the perfect situation, seems to correlate directly to the degree you need a daily wellness routine.

～　～　～

The progression of the following five sections is deliberately structured to open your breathing from the center out. We start by reviving the breath and getting the juices flowing. Next, we open the center of the body—the place where breathing is generated. Then we move on to releasing the lower channels in the body—the abdomen, lower back, and hips so that the breath can flow freely both into and from these areas. We then focus on releasing unnecessary tension in the secondary respiratory muscles. When the neck, shoulders, and upper back release we feel calm, which further elicits deep breathing. In the last section we take advantage of this new openness in the body by practicing deep relaxation, allowing life-giving energy to circulate into every cell.

WAKING UP THE BREATH

Tapping and Percussion

You'll Need

An optional helping partner

Purpose

The purpose of this exercise is to loosen any congestion in the lungs and to stimulate your breathing function. It is a wonderful way to perk up and wake up when you are feeling mental fatigue or lassitude. If you work in a sedentary job and get little exercise your lungs may be quite lethargic and your breathing muscles weak. This exercise is fun to do first thing in the morning next to an open window or, better yet, outside in the fresh air. Having a helping partner is especially nice, because they can get to those areas that are more difficult to reach. This exercise can also be done in a group, by forming a circle with everyone working on the person in front of them.

Here's How

Front of chest Make your hands into relaxed fists. Begin tapping the front of your chest, just below the collarbones, on and around the sternum (Figure 17). You should make it strong and steady but not painful. While you tap take five breaths in and out and on your fifth exhalation forcefully exhale the breath through the mouth with a "ha" sound. For added impact open the mouth wide, and with wide eyes throw your tongue out of your mouth like a lion (Figure 18). This is called Lion's Pose and it's wonderful for releasing tension in the jaw and throat. For an even greater release in the lungs I like to do a Tarzan roar on my exhalations. Sure to impress the neighbors, it also opens the throat and loosens the diaphragm. Repeat this five times, ending with an exhalation.

Lower ribs Now tap over the entire surface of your middle and lower ribs beneath the breasts. Let your tapping extend to the sides of the ribs as well. Repeat five rounds of five breaths each, throwing the breath out with a "ha" on the fifth exhalation.

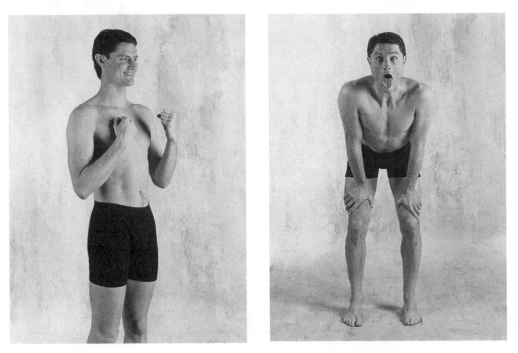

FIGURE 17   FIGURE 18

Back lungs If you have a partner have them tap on the upper back area around the tops of the shoulders as well as in the space between your spine and shoulder blades. Never bang on the spine itself. Repeat five rounds of five breaths, ending each round with a Lion's Pose exhalation.

Lower back lungs (kidney area) Bend your knees and reach around to tap the area just above your waist, either side of your spine. The lower part of the lungs can become quite stale if you breathe shallowly or predominantly with your chest. If you have a partner, brace your hands firmly on your thighs and let your friend tap away at your lower back lungs. Keep your breath moving, forcefully exhaling every five or so breaths.

Now stand and just let yourself observe your breathing and how you feel. Enjoy the tingling feeling throughout your skin and body. If this is the only breath work you are doing today, consider taking a brisk walk or enjoying a hot shower. The day is off to a good start.

Breath Stretches

Here's How

Breathing in to the Front Stand (or sit) with your feet hips-width apart. Clasp your hands behind your back and extend your arms down toward your heels. As you inhale, lift and open your chest and let your chin release down toward your chest. Feel the front lungs and chest inflating (Figure 19A). Exhale and release, coming back to the neutral standing position. Repeat this three times, directing your breath fully into the front of your chest.

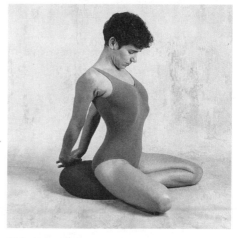

FIGURE 19A

Breathing in to the Back Clasp your left wrist with your right hand and extend the arms in front of your body. As you inhale, round your back and bend your knees so that your whole body is curling forward. Feel the back lungs inflating (Figure 19B). Exhale and release, coming back to the neutral standing position. Repeat this three times, directing your breath fully into the back part of your body.

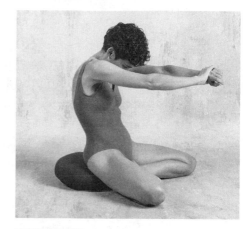

FIGURE 19B

Breathing in to the Sides Bring your right hand to rest on the right side of your rib cage just underneath your armpit. Extend the left arm down the outside of the left thigh. On an inhalation bend to the left side. Press your right hand firmly into your ribs and direct your breath to expand into the right side of the rib cage (Figure 19C). Exhale and return to the neutral position and repeat on the other side. Do three rounds on each side.

Now take a moment to stand and feel how your breath is moving. Notice if your breath is moving more strongly and whether you are more mentally

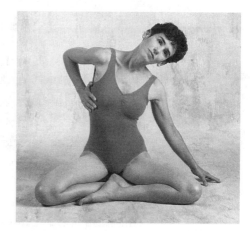

FIGURE 19C

alert. You are now ready to continue with the more specific body opening movements.

OPENING THE CENTER

Breathing is initiated centrally in the body, so this is where we must start to free the breathing process. The movements in this section focus on opening the torso and the spinal column.

Roll Downs

Purpose

I do this exercise almost every day and enjoy the overall feeling of release as it loosens the entire body as well as opening up each segment of the spinal column. I also use it as a diagnostic tool, feeling for the areas in my body that are sore or stiff so that I can pay extra attention to those parts later in my practice.

Here's How

In a standing position slowly let your head curl forward until your chin is resting on your chest (or as close to your chest as is comfortable without straining) (Figure 20A). Relax your jaw by opening your mouth and take a few breaths out through the mouth. After a few breaths you may begin to feel the pulse of the breath slightly lifting the head and neck up and down in a nodding motion. Once you feel this, follow the pulse of your breath, gradually rolling down through each segment of your spine. Let the weight of the head, chest, and arms gradually lengthen the spine. Generously bend your knees as you start to curl down through your upper back (Figure 20B) and continue to do this until you are hanging forward over bent knees. Take a few breaths at the bottom of the movement, checking that you are not holding any unnecessary tension in your neck around the base of the skull. Now press down through your feet, and using this downward pressure through your legs (rather than making your back muscles lift you), begin to curl back to standing. Check that you are not lifting up the head and neck during this movement, (Figure 20—incorrect). When you keep the head and neck relaxed their weight will give your entire spine a stretch.

FIGURE 20A

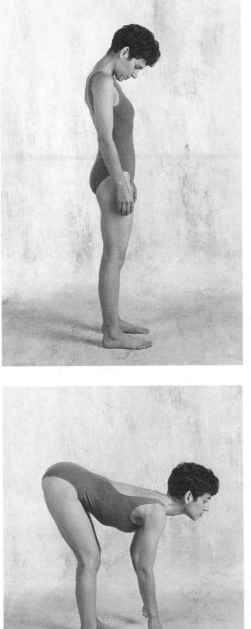

FIGURE 20B

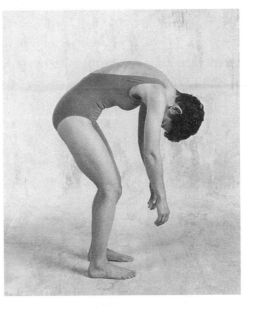

FIGURE 20 Incorrect

FIGURE 20C

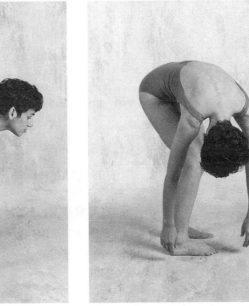

Now turn your head to look over your right shoulder and down along the side of your right thigh. Slowly curl down, this time bending to the side so that you end up with your body draped over the outside of your right leg. Make sure you let your knees bend and that both arms drape to the right side (Figure 20C). Although your spine will be twisting to the side you should try to keep your knees parallel rather than letting them turn inwards. Push down through your feet to come back up to standing, being careful to relax your neck and shoulders so that they are the last part of you to come upright. Repeat the same movement to the left side.

Now do the whole series, center, right, and left, another two times, concentrating on synchronizing the movement of your knees so that they are fully bent when you are at the bottom of the movement and so that they just straighten when your head comes upright. Your knees will then be in a constant, fluid motion. The third time you do the roll downs, give the areas in your spine that feel tight or sore extra attention by moving very slowly through those segments.

The Cat

Purpose

Because the breath arises from the central torso, any stiffness in the center of the body will limit the generation of the breath. If the spine is rigid it can act like a stiff rod running the length of the torso, stifling the natural rise and fall of the breath. When flexible, the spine can move like a rolling wave. In this exercise we start to differentiate the movements along the length of the spine to free up the center. Notice your breath before you begin and then check it again when you've completed both parts.

Here's How

The Cat, Variation A Come onto all fours with your hands directly under your shoulders and your knees underneath your hips. Feel how your breath is moving. Begin by rounding your back upwards, drawing your tail towards your head as you look back at your crotch (Figure 21A). Then relax and let the spine curve the other way, raising the head and tailbone into the air, creating a gentle arch in the back (Figure 21B). Continue slowly flexing and extending, allowing the breath to synchronize itself with both movements. When does it feel good

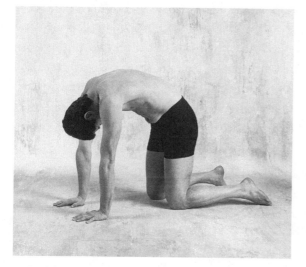

FIGURE 21A

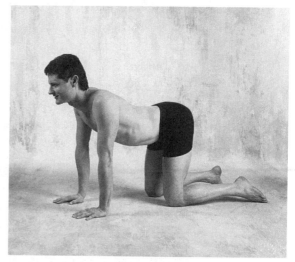

FIGURE 21B

to inhale? When to exhale? Don't try to impose a specific pattern but allow the breath to emerge. When you have done about ten rounds, rest with your buttocks on your heels, allowing your head and arms to relax on the floor.

   The Cat, Variation B Now return to the all–fours position. This time you are going to work on one small segment of your back at a time. Imagine that you are a kitten being picked up by your fur. Start with the uppermost part of your back where the neck joins the torso. As you breathe in strongly push upwards in this one spot, pressing down through your arms to get the optimum lift. Imagine that you are being lifted right from that point and that you are directing your breath into that area. As you exhale, let your vertebrae release the other way, allowing that very same part of the back to depress downward. When you release, let go of any tension in the back rather than trying to push the spine lower. Continue down the spine a few vertebrae at a time until you reach the place where your lumbar vertebrae join the sacrum (about where the line of your underpants would be). When you are through take a moment to feel how your breath is moving throughout your body. Also make a mental note of any areas in your spine where you felt restriction or stiffness. If you repeat this exercise you might want to spend a little more time on these places. Now rest, bringing your buttocks onto your heels, relaxing the head and arms on the floor.

Variation—Working with a Partner The exercise above can be very powerful if done with the help of a partner. Instead of getting on all-fours you will interlock your hands and bring the elbows to the floor directly underneath the shoulders and the knees underneath the hips. Your partner will assist you by pressing down on the place you wish to open, allowing you to focus more precisely on each area. They will also be making you work against some resistance. The helper can kneel facing their partner's back, or in any other position where he can effectively put the weight of his body behind the movement. The helping partner crosses his thumbs and places them on either side of the spine, but not directly on the bones (Figure 22A).

Start at the level of the spine that corresponds to the tops of the shoulder blades. (Do not press on the neck vertebrae as this can injure the spine.) The helping partner presses firmly downwards so you will have to work more strongly to lift that part of your back with your breath. As you inhale and round upward against the pressure of your partner's thumbs, direct the breath into that area (Figure 22B). As you exhale, let the spine release the other way (Figure 22C). Your partner should keep his pressure consistent during both the flexion and the extension part of the movement. After a few repetitions, the helping

FIGURE 22A

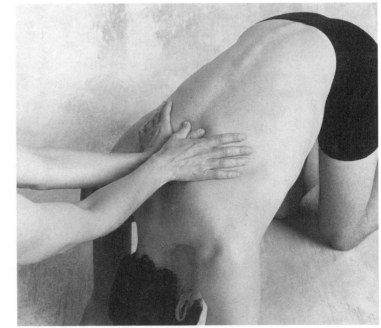

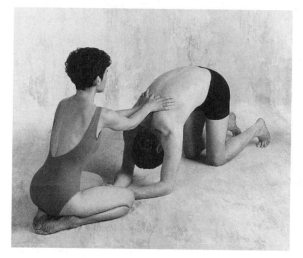

FIGURE 22B

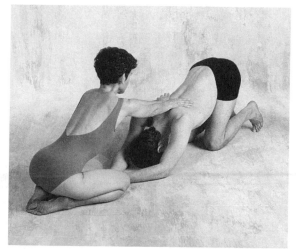

FIGURE 22C

partner moves up to the next segment and continues segment by segment until he is finally just above the crack of the buttocks.

As your partner moves his hands down your spine you should direct your breath into each specific area. Most people find that inhaling and flexing and exhaling during the release is most effective, but experiment to find what feels right for you. You may notice places that feel particularly tight. Let your partner know that you'd like to spend a little more time in those tight spots. Take four or five breaths in and out in each of these areas, until you can feel your back moving more freely. Your helper may also notice places where the skin and muscle feel glued together or where the tissue feels calloused, dry, or leathery. They can encourage you to give special emphasis to those areas that are lacking in circulation. If at any time you feel tired, take a rest break before continuing onto the next segment. When you are finished, take a moment to sit in a kneeling position and to feel how your breath is moving.

OPENING THE LOWER CHANNELS

When we can't move freely in the lower body we tend to compensate by breathing higher up with the secondary respiratory muscles in the neck, shoulders, and back. In this section we focus on freeing the pelvis, hips, lower back, and belly so that the wave of the breath is unimpeded. As this surge becomes stronger, the breath can move from the center of the body into the periphery, radiating out like a star's light to all our limbs.

Pelvic and Hip Openers

You'll Need

A tie or belt

Purpose

During full breathing there is a natural oscillation of the pelvis around the hips (see Illustrations 1 and 2). Through inactivity or unnecessary holding patterns, the muscles in the hips and lower back can freeze, preventing this natural oscillation from happening. In this exercise we focus on loosening the hip joints, opening through the pelvic floor and releasing the legs. Check in with your breathing before you begin and afterwards.

Here's How

Lie down in the Effortless Rest position (see Figure 3). Take a moment just to feel your breath moving through your abdomen and through your pelvic diaphragm. Notice how your pelvis rocks ever so slightly to and fro with each breath cycle. On your next exhalation allow the right knee to come into your chest and with both hands take hold of your shin just below the knee. As you breathe in allow the leg to move away from you (Figure 23A) and as you breathe out invite the leg closer toward the chest (Figure 23B). Follow the lead of the breath as you draw the leg in toward you, bending the elbows, and then as you let the leg move out by slightly straightening the arms. These movements needn't be large, and in fact, the smaller they are the more easily you will be able to feel the oscillating action of the pelvis. Continue for a few minutes, noticing how the spine alternately extends and flexes with the pelvis. Then let your leg come back to the starting position. Now repeat the movement on the left side.

When you have done both sides you are ready to continue with the deeper leg releases. Let your right leg come into your chest again and place a tie or belt around the sole of your foot. Slowly extend the leg until it is straight (Figure 23C). Feel

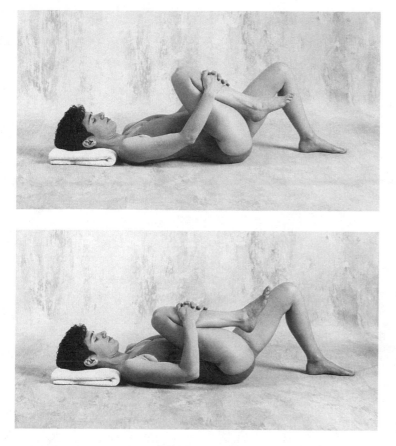

FIGURE 23A

FIGURE 23B

the muscles along the back of the leg and find the place where the stretching sensation captures your attention but is not so intense that you would rather be somewhere else! Let your breath descend down into the lower abdomen and imagine it moving all the way into your thigh. Instead of pulling the leg toward you and forcing the opening, wait until you feel a "giving" moment when the muscles soften and release. This is your cue to *invite* the leg to come closer to the chest. Continue for up to 3 minutes, breathing, relaxing, and patiently waiting for an opening moment before drawing the leg closer to you.

Now turn the leg out 45 degrees and open it to the side; allow the other leg to open and counter balance this action. Your legs will be like an open book with your torso as the spine (Figure 23D). Feel the opening coming all the way from the pelvic floor, from your genitals and anal area into the inner thighs and down to the inner ankles. Keep your abdomen centered so that your naval faces

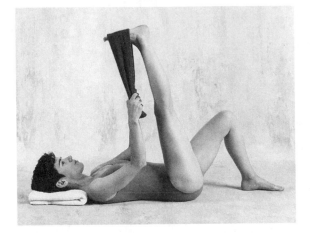

FIGURE 23C

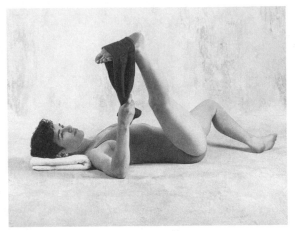

FIGURE 23D

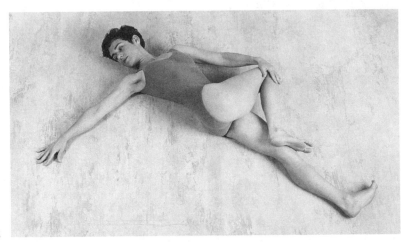

FIGURE 23E

the sky. This will keep the action focused in the hips. Stay for a minute or so and then bring the right leg back up to the perpendicular position on an exhalation.

For the final opening, release the tie from around the foot. Bend your right knee and slowly cross it over to the left and onto the floor (if the knee doesn't come to the floor, support it with a pillow). Counter the movement by extending the right arm along the floor in line with the shoulder. You will feel a strong stretch along the outside of your hip and buttock area. You can intensify the opening by pressing down on the outside of the right knee with your left hand (Figure 23E). Continue to let your breath move deeply into the abdominal area, drawing the right leg deeper into the movement on your exhalations. After a minute release the stretch, rolling back onto your spine and returning to the Effortless Rest position. Just for fun, take a little walk around the room to feel the difference between your left and right side. Your right and left sides may feel like two entirely different personalities. Take a moment to relax and then do the entire sequence with the other leg.

When you are through doing both sides, lie on your back in the Effortless Rest position and draw both knees into the chest. Hold your knees firmly with both hands and see if you can feel the rocking motion of the pelvis as you breathe in and out. Notice how the expansion in the abdomen draws the pelvis into slight extension causing the lower back to lift away from the floor and how the retraction of the exhalation causes the spine to flatten towards the floor. After opening your hips it will be easier to feel the way the pelvis moves with the breath. If you still cannot perceive any movement, don't despair. Most people can feel this pelvic movement within a few days of working on the exercise.

Revolved Belly Pose

Purpose

This posture loosens and releases congestion throughout the abdominal area, and opens the sides of the diaphragm and the intercostal muscles in between the ribs. The posture also stimulates the function of the abdominal organs by alternately squeezing and releasing them like sponges. When you release the twist, new fluids rush into the tissues and organs, drenching them with fresh oxygenated blood.

Here's How

Lie in the Effortless Rest position with your arms extended out to the sides in line with your shoulders. Become aware of your breath moving in the abdomen. Now lift your buttocks off the floor and shift it about 6 inches off-center to the left. This maneuver will ensure that your spine is in a neutral position when you later twist to the side. Bring your legs towards your chest one at a time. On an exhalation let your knees slowly lower to the right side on the floor (or onto a pillow if bringing them to the floor is too difficult). Extend your awareness back through the opposite arm and the chest so that you feel a long diagonal opening

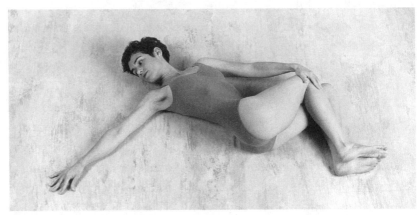

FIGURE 24

through the body (Figure 24). Spend a minute or two allowing the fullness of the breath to rock the body, letting your abdomen be contentedly loose. As the body releases you will find that the whole lower back and pelvis as well as the rest of the spine move clearly with each phase of the breath cycle. Celebrate any movements that you can feel, however small, and open into the pleasure of the body releasing. When you are ready, let your knees fold back into your chest, and then roll onto your spine before continuing on to the other side.

If you feel so uncomfortable that you can't relax into the movement, try doing *brief* repetitions of 10 seconds on each side. After three rounds try staying for 1 minute. The brief stays serve to progressively loosen the muscles without building intensity. You can also place two pillows either side of you so that your knees do not have to come all the way to the floor. This is a particularly good way to work if you are recovering from a back injury.

Supported Bound Angle

You'll Need

> At least 3 blankets and 2 pillows or a breathing bolster (See Resources)
> A dark cloth or eye bag to cover the eyes (See Resources)

Purpose

> Since they are the seat of our sexual energy, the soft abdomen, the genital and anal areas, as well as the inner thighs are all very sensitive and vulnerable places.

These are places where we tend to store strong emotions. Whether we have experienced self-consciousness, shame, or ecstasy from our loins, it is not unusual to feel a hesitancy to open fully here. Full body breathing depends on being able to relax and release these intimate areas. In this pose you can let gravity do the work of opening and releasing so that you can completely relax. It is a particularly nourishing posture for women during menstruation and before childbirth because it increases circulation and alleviates cramps. If practiced while more than 3 months pregnant the torso should be elevated at a 45 degree angle to prevent compression of the blood flow to both mother and fetus.

Here's How

Fold 2–3 blankets so that they form a rectangular bolster about 8 inches wide, 4 inches high and at least 3 feet long, or use a breathing bolster. Sit with your buttocks on the floor directly in front of the bolster and bring the soles of your feet together so that your legs form a diamond shape. Reclining back onto your elbows, lie back onto the bolster being careful to center your spine. Place a pillow underneath each thigh so that your legs are fully supported and you do not feel any pulling in your inner groin, thighs, or hips. Raise your head slightly on a folded towel so that your forehead is a little higher than your chin and then release your shoulders back so that your arms extend with the palms up (Figure 25). From this position let the weight of gravity release your hips and inner

FIGURE 25

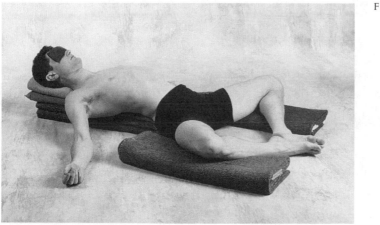

thighs. Focus your attention on the abdomen and in through the pelvic floor, softening and relaxing with each breath cycle. If the room is cool cover yourself with a blanket so that you will be warm throughout your relaxation. Stay for 3–10 minutes, resting with your eyes closed. You can increase the depth of your relaxation by covering the eyes with a dark cloth or eye bag. If you are experiencing menstrual cramps you can place a weight such as a sandbag (see Resources) across your lower abdomen. When you are ready to come out, use your hands to raise one knee and roll over onto your side. Take a few moments to collect yourself before sitting up. Take a brief walk to feel the difference in your lower body.

OPENING THE UPPER CHANNELS

It's rare to meet anyone these days who doesn't feel upper back, neck, and shoulder tension. Much of this tension is caused by overusing the secondary respiratory muscles during chest breathing and hyperventilation. In this section we focus on releasing these overused muscles.

Shoulder Clock

You'll Need

A wall

Purpose

When we've become accustomed to breathing high in the body the secondary respiratory muscles in the chest, neck, and shoulders become chronically tight. In chest breathing the shoulders lift up and down. As a result the trapezius muscles along the tops of the shoulder can become like tightropes that over time come to feel normal, albeit an awful kind of "normal." This simple exercise is a wonderful way to release the front, side, and back of the shoulder so that the shoulders once again release down away from the ears. The Shoulder Clock is especially good for those who have arthritis in these areas.

Here's How

Stand at a right angle to a wall with your right shoulder facing the wall. Check first that your feet are hips-width apart so you'll have a solid foundation underneath you. Stand about 8 inches away from the wall. Depending on your flexibility you can move closer to the wall, which will make the exercise more challenging, or as far away as a foot or more, which will make it easier. Extend your arm up the wall like the hand of a clock pointing to twelve o'clock. Take a moment to press down through your heels and to relax your neck and jaw. After several breath cycles, extend the arm back to one o'clock (Figure 26). Keep reaching the arm as high as you can up the wall. Again stay for several breaths and continue moving through the imaginary digits of the clock face until you reach three o'clock. As you come to three o'clock, lean your chest forward, slightly turning your breastbone toward the center of the room. You'll feel a strong opening in the front of your chest and shoulder, an area that can become chronically tight during upper chest breathing. Take several breaths here and then let your arm swing down to your side. Stand for a moment and feel the dif-

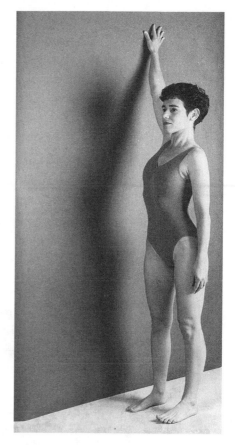

FIGURE 26

ference between the two arms. If you look in a mirror or have a friend look at you, you may be able to see that one arm is longer than the other. The extra length is simply a measure of how much you have released the shoulder downwards. Can you feel which side of your chest is breathing more fully?

Repeat the shoulder clock on the other side. If you have time, return to the first side and do the exercise standing a little closer to the wall.

Shoulder and Upper Back Release

You'll Need

A chair

Purpose

The upper back and shoulders can also become chronically tight when we rely too much on the secondary respiratory muscles. The shoulders begin to round forward and down, the chest collapses inwards, and the spine develops an exaggerated thoracic curvature (known in medical terminology as a *kyphosis*). This is the posturing normal to a sudden fight or flight response, as when we hear a loud sound or duck to avoid being hit by someone. Then again, it can become an unconscious way of holding ourselves all the time. Caving in through the front of the body compresses the diaphragm, making full breathing impossible. By opening through the upper chest, shoulders, and back the energy we once used to contract and withdraw from life is given over to expanding and engaging life.

Here's How

Place a chair against the wall with the seat facing you. Come into a kneeling position in front of the chair, and place your elbows shoulder-width apart on the edge of the chair. Let the weight rest on the *outer* edge of your elbows, rather than the inner edge so that your shoulder girdle broadens out to the sides. Rest your forehead on the edge of the chair and press the fingertips together over your head in a "prayer" position. Walk your knees back until they are directly under your hips (Figure 27). Expand your breath into your upper chest, back,

FIGURE 27

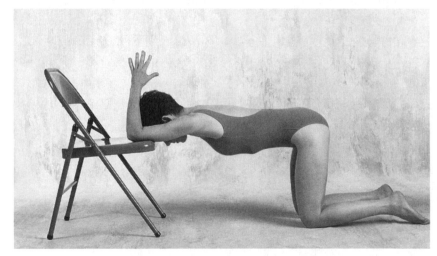

and shoulders, pressing the elbows firmly downward, as you reach back through your hips. Feel the armpits lengthening and with each breath allow the upper back to release downwards. Stay for as long as you feel comfortable, gradually deepening the intensity of the opening. When you've had enough, slowly walk your knees in towards your arms until you can take your elbows off the chair. Rest for a few moments in a kneeling position enjoying the sensation of the upper body opening to the breath.

Gateway Pose

You'll Need

A thick blanket or exercise mat, a wall for the variation.

Purpose

This posture allows you to achieve a deep opening in the intercostal muscles that lie between the ribs. These primary respiratory muscles are responsible for both inhalation and exhalation. Unfortunately, there are very few movements that we do in our everyday activities that thoroughly stretch these unsung heroes of the breath. Unlike many other muscles in the body, once the intercostal muscles are released they tend to stay that way. Because your breathing deepens with their increased length, the fuller breathing provides an ongoing massage that sustains the initial stretch.

Here's How

Come into a kneeling position with your knees well padded by a thick blanket. Now bring your buttocks up off your heels so that you are standing on your knees with your body in one line from your head to your knees. Turn your right leg out and extend the leg out to the side, so your foot is in line with your shoulder. Flex the toes of the right foot. Now extend your left arm over your head and slowly begin to bend over your right leg, letting your right arm slide down the length of the leg as you do so (Figure 28). Move with your breath, releasing and lengthening further on your exhalations. Sustain this position for 5–10 breaths before coming up and over to the other side. Repeat the movement twice to each side, going a little further, if you can, the second time.

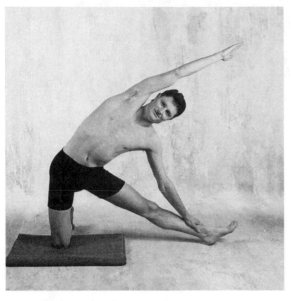

FIGURE 28

Variation

In this variation you'll use a wall to intensify the stretch. Place yourself so that the foot of the extended leg is pressed against a wall, with the heel of the foot on the floor and the sole flat against the wall. Now as you bend to the side, let the upper arm come to touch the wall. Press the fingers into the wall and begin to turn the chest up toward the sky. The pressure of the fingers against the wall will intensify the sensation along the sides of the ribs as well as your flanks. Using your breath to help you release the muscles on the exhalation, bring the hand further down the wall until you have reached your threshold. Stay there for a few deep breaths, letting the body oscillate slightly into and out of the movement. Release and take the second side.

When you return to the kneeling position take a moment to notice how your breath feels before continuing.

Diaphragm Release

You'll Need

A few blankets or a Yoga Bolster (see Resources)

Purpose

Most of our everyday activities involve bending forward and everything from sitting in chairs, to working at computers, to washing dishes, to making beds compress the front of the body. Over time the upper back can become rounded, narrowing the chest and making full breathing virtually impossible. The following movements are designed to release tension in the spine while liberating the chest and diaphragmatic muscles.

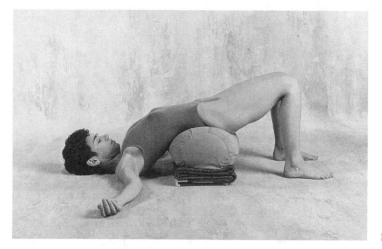

FIGURE 29A

Variation A

Take a few firm blankets and roll them into a tight cylinder about 10 inches in diameter and about 3 feet in length (or use a Yoga Bolster—see Resources). Sit on the blankets or bolster and slowly recline back, first onto your elbows and then onto your upper back and shoulders so that your buttocks are atop the bolster. Your head, neck, upper back, and shoulders will be resting on the floor (Figure 29A). Keep your knees bent as you remain in this reclined backbend. Notice in this position that your lower ribs and indentation below the sternum are quite pronounced. This is where the diaphragm is located. In this gentle backbend you can allow the diaphragm to release, broadening and lengthening at the same time. As you stay in the position focus on relaxing the abdomen and letting go of any unnecessary tension in your shoulders. Stay for up to 5 minutes and then roll over onto your side before sitting up.

Variation B

Sit on the floor with your knees bent and your bolster directly behind you. Bring your elbows to rest on the bolster and slowly recline over the bolster so that it crosses your body at the level of your nipples (mid–shoulder blades). Your neck, head, and shoulders will be on the floor on one side of the bolster and your buttocks and legs will be resting on the other. If you cannot release the shoulders onto the floor without creating an uncomfortable arch in your neck you proba-

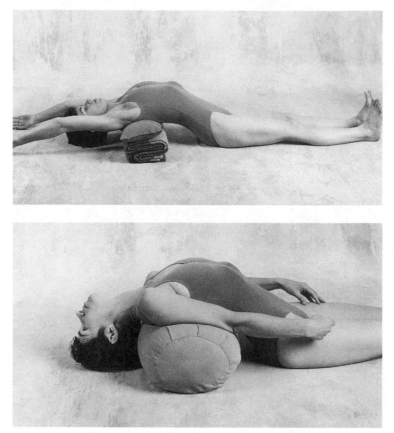

FIGURE 29B

FIGURE 29C

bly need to reduce the diameter of the bolster (try about 6 inches), or alternatively place a small pillow under your head to reduce the angle of the head. (In Figure 29C the bolster is too big, causing the head and neck to overarch. This can also be caused by not moving far enough over the bolster.) Allow your arms to relax over your head with the elbows bent. Stay here for about a minute, letting the body become accustomed to the opening. If you would like to increase the intensity of the opening, extend your arms over your head along the floor. At the same time you can extend the legs until they are completely straight (Figure 29B). In this final position, the front of the diaphragm receives a strong opening. As you stay in the pose, focus on relaxing the muscles in your upper back and chest and allowing the breath to expand there. After you have stayed in the pose for a few minutes feel free to experiment with your positioning by placing the bolster a little higher or lower on your back. Rather than move the bolster, it is better to bend your knees and scoot headward or footward before lying back again.

This stretch can be very intense the first time, so don't stay too long. When you're ready to come out, bend your knees and roll onto your side. Never try to come out of the position by directly sitting up. Relax on your side before coming to a sitting position. Once seated, close the eyes and feel the quality of your breathing.

DEEP RELAXATION

Helpful Hints Before You Begin

Covering the eyes with an eye bag (see Resources), eye mask, or scarf will aid you immeasurably during relaxation. Covering the eyes eliminates visual distractions and relaxes the muscles around the eyes. Another technique which I have found amazingly effective, is to *lightly* wind a soft cotton ace ba ndage around the head so that it covers the eyes, forehead, and temples. The bandage should not pull on the skin around the eyes. The gentle pressure of the bandage against the frontalis and temporal muscles induces an immediate and deep state of relaxation. It does look funny (my students call it the "post–brain surgery" look), but it is so effective I gladly accept the teasing. After only 15 minutes of having the eyes covered, deep lines and furrows begin to uncrease and the face looks revived and youthful.

The Waterfall

You'll Need

3 blankets or a yoga bolster (see Resources)

Purpose

This restorative posture is pure ambrosia for the over-worked nervous system. Whenever the body is turned upside-down the diaphragm is put in a position where it is easier to exhale. Normally the diaphragm has to work against gravity to ascend during the exhalation. When we invert the body, gravity is now assisting full exhalation and as a result the inhalation naturally starts to lengthen and deepen. At the same time the heart rate slows down and the blood pressure decreases. As the breath deepens the body receives a message that all is well and the positive feedback loop of this good news draws us into a deeper and deeper state of relaxation.

This supported backbend also opens the spine, chest, and diaphragm. Blood is drained from the legs, directing it into the abdomen, chest, and throat areas where it can bathe the sex, thymus, and thyroid glands. The inversion of the torso also helps to drain excess fluid and congestion from the lungs, which can help those with chronic asthma and bronchitis to clear their air passages. This is an excellent posture for those with fatigue and those recovering from illness. Next time you have the impulse to take a nap or raid the refrigerator for an energy boost, instead try practicing the Waterfall for 10–15 minutes.

Here's How

Fold the blankets so they form a rectangular bolster about 6–10 inches high, about 10 inches wide and at least 3 feet long. People who are very flexible or who have long torsos should have a higher and slighter wider prop. Place the bolster lengthwise along a wall, leaving about a 2-inch gap between the bolster and the wall.

Sit on one end of the bolster and carefully roll onto your side so that your right hip is supported on the bolster and your right shoulder is on the floor (Figure 30A). Using your right arm for support, roll your body so that your buttocks are on the bolster with your legs extended straight up the wall, and your shoulders, head, and neck resting on the floor. Your chin will be drawn slightly down towards your chest. In the final position your hips will be very close if not touching the wall, your abdomen will be parallel to the floor, and the chest and spine will cascade over the bolster (Figure 30B). Imagine the pose like a waterfall: the legs are the first waterfall, with fluid pooling in the basin of the abdomen, the chest and spine are the second waterfall, with fluid pooling in the throat and upper chest.

If you do not find the position comfortable experiment with the height and with the width of the propping. People with very long or short torsos may need to adjust the propping to accommodate their dimensions. Still others may find that it feels better when the blankets are stacked either lower or higher. The

FIGURE 30B

FIGURE 30A

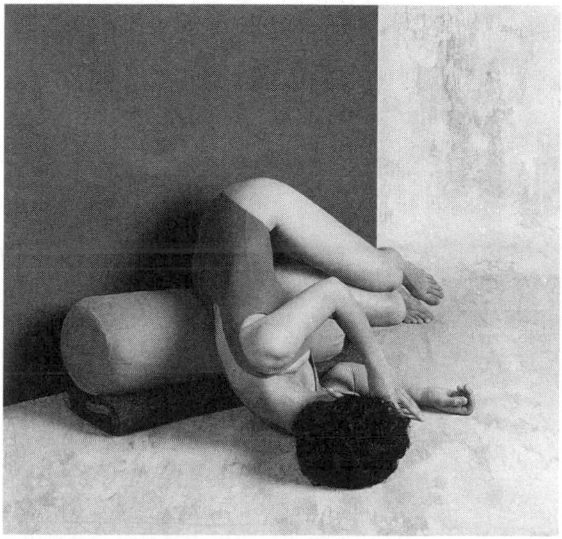

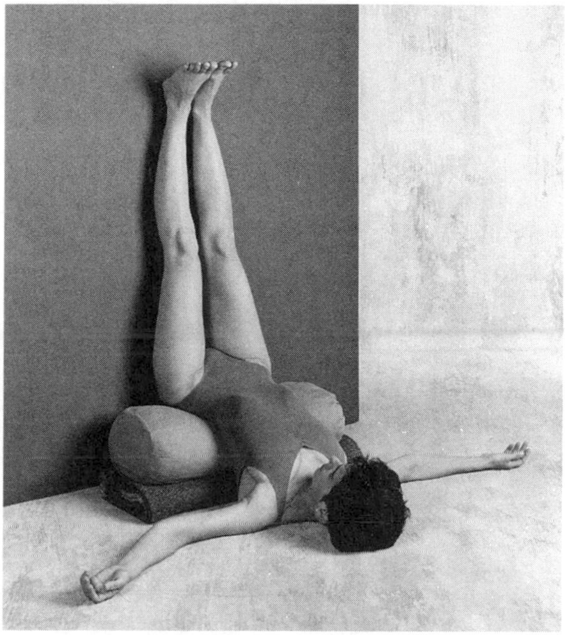

small investment of time required is insignificant compared to the Waterfall's powerful restorative effect. When you get it right it should feel like you could fall asleep in the position.

Once you are set, close your eyes (or cover your eyes with an eye bag or scarf) and relax completely for 5–15 minutes. Observe the change in your breathing without trying to manipulate it in any way. Many people report a sensation of the breath spontaneously opening as their mind becomes quiet. One student described this shift as "the mind collapsing." You can help promote this by visualizing the brain as a balloon gradually receding away from the inner skull with each exhalation. If other calming images arise use these to lure yourself into relaxation.

When you are ready to come out, either roll onto your side and off the bolster, or bend your knees and push yourself away from the wall until you are lying flat on the floor. Take a moment to let your body adjust before you sit up.

Cautions:

- People with glaucoma, detached retina, or high blood pressure should not practice this pose.

- Pregnant woman should not practice this pose after the third month of pregnancy.
- People with acute neck injuries should avoid this pose.

Supported Child's Pose

You'll Need

A stack of blankets or 3–4 pillows

Purpose

This is a very soothing posture that helps to elicit both deep abdominal breathing and full movement of the breath throughout the whole body. This position also comforts the soft organs in the throat, belly, and genitals, thus creating a deep feeling of safety and security, much as a child would feel pressed close to the mother. For these reasons this pose is very helpful for people who feel themselves to be in a chronic state of anxiety and tension. It is also good for those people who do not find it relaxing to lie on their back. I personally practice the supported child's pose when I am traveling to mitigate some of the woozy effects of jet lag. This is also an excellent pose for women with menstrual cramps and can be made even more effective if a folded towel is placed underneath the abdomen to provide deep pressure to the belly.

When in doubt, hit horizontal!

Here's How

Stack the pillows one on top of the other, or fold your blankets to the size of a pillow. Lie belly down straddling the pillows, with your arms and legs draped over the sides. Stagger the pillows to form a stair step so that the head and neck can release downwards onto the pillow below (Figure 31).

This pose is especially nice when done in bed, with the cushioning of a mattress under the knees. As you lie, notice how the breath begins to deepen in the abdomen and throughout the back of your body. As you feel your breath deepen, relax your jaw and open your mouth, letting out a few deep sighs. With each exhalation let the arms and legs become heavier and heavier until there is no tension in the hips and knees or in the upper back or shoulders. Stay as long

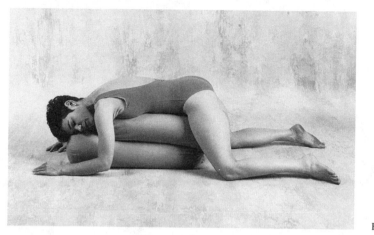

FIGURE 31

as you feel comfortable and when you are ready use your arms to help yourself up to a sitting position.

You can also do a variation of this position by lying belly down on a soft surface. The same response is elicited here, but it is less relaxing for the hips and legs, and may be uncomfortable in the neck if you stay for more than a few minutes.

Breathing Easy Position

You'll Need

2–4 blankets (or more if you are pregnant) or a breathing bolster (see Resources)

Purpose

From a prone position, raising the head and chest slightly above the height of the abdomen makes it easier for the diaphragm to move freely. This position can be used for your guided relaxations or for the breathing inquiries in chapter 6. It is also an excellent position for clearing the breathing passages when the lungs or sinuses are congested because of colds and flus. After the third month of pregnancy, women will find that this elevated position affords them more room to breathe as the baby grows larger. It also will not endanger the baby by interrupting the flow of blood to the fetus as can happen in completely supine positions.

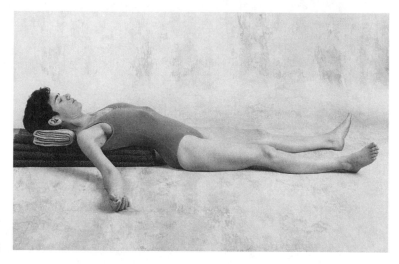

FIGURE 32

As your pregnancy progresses, increase the angle of incline up to 45 degrees until you feel a release around your diaphragm area.

Here's How

Fold the blankets into a bolster about 3 inches high, 8–10 inches wide, and at least 3 feet long. Lie with your buttocks on the floor and slowly recline back being careful that your spine is symmetrical along the length of the bolster. Bend your knees and lift the pelvis briefly, drawing the buttocks under so that the lower back is long and released. Then extend the legs straight letting them relax about a foot apart. Raise the head with a folded towel until the forehead is slightly higher than the chin (Figure 32).

You can now use this position to do the following guided relaxations or as a starting point for the breathing inquiries in chapter 6.

Guided Deep Relaxation

You'll Need

A warm, quiet place
A blanket to cover you
A small pillow for under your head
2–4 blankets, if you want to do the Breathing Easy position.

Purpose

Once we have forgotten what it feels like to be completely relaxed it becomes increasingly difficult to recognize when we are holding tension. Learning how to enter a deep yet attentive state of relaxation can establish a familiar baseline that we can return to over and over again. As awareness is honed, we can recognize tension states *before* they arise.

There are many different ways to enter a deep state of relaxation. The following are three guided relaxation sessions that you can explore. In all the relaxation sessions prepare as follows:

Begin by lying down on a soft surface making sure that the surface beneath you is warm and that your body is symmetrical on the floor. Take a moment to look down your body to check that your head, breastbone, pubic bone, and the space between your feet are in one line. Place a folded towel or a small pillow under your head and neck so that your forehead is slightly higher than your chin. Lastly cover yourself with a blanket so that you will feel warm and secure. (Alternatively, assume the Breathing Easy position.)

Following the Lure of the Breath

As you lie on the floor take a moment to settle, feeling the weight of your body surrendering to the floor. Scan your body for tension, beginning with the head. Soften the skin across your forehead and let the skin become smooth. Sense into the muscles around the eyes, letting any tension there dissolve with the out-going breath. Let the jaw fall open and release the temples back toward the ears. Allow the lips to part slightly, relaxing the tongue and all the muscles around your lips. Feel down into your throat, taking a moment to swallow a few times to relax any constriction in this area. As you open the throat, let your exhalation pass out through your mouth for a few breaths, sighing as you do so. Continue in this way slowly down through your body, inviting each part of yourself to relax and open.

When you feel settled draw your attention to your breath. Listen to the sound of the breath and feel the sensation of the breath. As you perceive the breath, let the sound or sensation of it draw you inward like the most tantalizing lure. This listening to the breath has the same quality of rapt attention that you have when you strain to hear a sonorous melody far off in the distance. Let the breath lure you back toward yourself.

Follow each breath as it arises and each breath as it passes away. Sense the first perceptible moment of the incoming breath and sense the very last whispers of the outgoing breath. Watch your breath as you might watch the waves of the ocean, endlessly arising, endlessly descending, changing from moment to moment. Now deep, now shallow, now long, now short, now smooth, now uneven. Follow the way that the breath changes from moment to moment.

Begin to focus more of your attention on the exhalation. Allow your mind to glide down the length of an exhalation to the very last whisper of the breath. Let the exhalation lure you down into the dark, quiet well of your being. Perceive the pause, however brief. With each successive exhalation let your attention rest more deeply on the pause at the end of the outgoing breath. This is the origin of the breath, where the breath arises and where the breath returns to. Let your entire being fall back into the pause, trusting that the new breath will arise without any effort on your part. As you surrender to the pause it will become longer and more spacious.

Do you tend to grab for the inhalation before it is ready to arise of its own accord? Can you simply allow the next breath to arise without effort? Does it surprise you how long the pause can become before you feel any desire to breathe in?

As you feel yourself entering a deep state of relaxation, let go of even the effort of following the lure of the breath and become the breath itself. "It" breathes you! Know that you can use the lure of your breath to return to yourself at any time and in any situation. Your breath is an ever-present resource that you can always draw from for rest and replenishment.

VI

Breathing Deeper

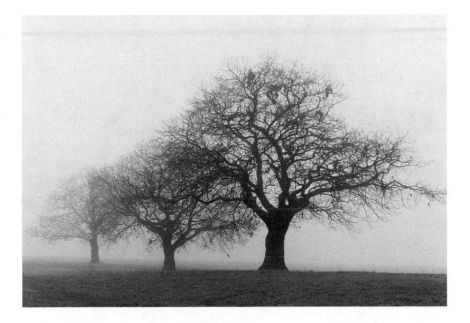

Time is Breath

—G. I. GURDJIEFF

*E*very time a musician plays a stringed instrument, he begins by tuning the strings. And just as a guitar can stay in tune for hours after having the strings adjusted, the rhythm, depth, and rate of your breathing can be altered for hours and even days after doing conscious breath work. When you do a breathing exercise you are enacting a "tuning" ritual. This tuning process can take as long as an hour or be as brief as one long exhalation. Combining focused breath work sessions with more casual "mini-breath checks" throughout the day, can, over time, completely alter the way in which you function, physically, mentally, and emotionally.

The purpose of doing breathing inquiries is not to learn how to take grand, dramatic breaths. This is a popular misconception that results in a great deal of ineffective huffing and puffing. It is not the flute player with the biggest breath that makes the best music, but the one who has smooth control of her breath. Similarly, the focus in all of the following exercises is on improving the quality of your breathing. These exercises will help to strengthen the muscles that support breathing, gradually enhancing their flexibility and resilience. Like any other muscle in the body, the diaphragm and the other primary respiratory muscles can become weak and tight. When you do breath work you are retraining your muscles to become strong and flexible and to move smoothly. You are also resetting the rhythm and rate of your breathing. As you change the way you breathe the carbon dioxide content of your blood changes, your neurological responses shift, and your endocrine levels undergo radical alteration. The respiratory centers in the lower brain stem respond to these changes by resetting themselves.

The respiratory control center is located in the medulla oblongata of the lower brain stem. It is extremely sensitive to changes in carbon dioxide (CO_2) levels in your blood and is therefore called a chemosensitive area. This control center is a part of your nervous system and it regulates the basic rhythm of your breathing. You also have chemoreceptors, the carotid bodies (in the neck), and aortic bodies (in the upper chest), which are also sensitive to CO_2 and O_2 levels in the blood. If there is even a slight increase or decrease of CO_2 both the chemosensitive area in the medulla, and the chemoreceptors in the carotid and aortic sinuses respond quickly. Their signals increase or decrease the rate of your breathing and thus the respiratory muscles are asked to speed up or slow down. Normally this happens outside our control, but because breathing can be consciously altered through the activity of the thinking brain (the cerebral cortex) or the limbic brain (the seat of the emotions) we can reset the "metronome" of our breathing at will. If we have had the habit of breathing too fast, the respiratory center resets itself to accommodate this accelerated pattern, and not always for our own good. There is also growing evidence to show that those who regularly meditate (a practice that is almost always accompanied by a reduced rate of breathing) have a decreased sensitivity to carbon dioxide.[1] So when you do breathing exercises you are actually changing the chemical and neurological systems that calibrate the entire breathing mechanism.

These breathing exercises are best done after opening the body with a few stretches or releasing movements, which you can choose from the previous chapter. I like to practice my breathing inquiries after doing a quiet sitting meditation, or after a deep relaxation in a reclining position. Because I tend to hyperventilate and chest breathe, I focus my attention on slowing down and breathing low. I am always amazed at how even 5 minutes of such practice can radically alter my breathing, and subsequently the way I feel for the rest of the day. Throughout the day I continue to have a glancing awareness of my breathing, consciously watching if my breathing speeds up for no good reason, or if I am holding my breath in any way. Over the last few years of doing breath work I've seen a great improvement in my health, my work performance, and most noticeable (to myself and to others), my ability to remain calm and centered in situations that would have seriously upset my equilibrium in the past.

Depending on what you've observed in the previous inquiries, tailor the exercises to your own needs. If you've been a chest or a collapsed breather and find that your diaphragmatic muscles are weak, spend more time on the diaphragmatic strengthening exercises, making sure that you relax the irrelevant secondary muscles as you do so. If you are a chronic hyperventilator, or someone who never exhales completely, use the exercises that focus on lengthening the exhalation and relaxing. If your breathing tends to be very erratic, experiment with the alternate nostril breathing.

It's completely normal to meet resistance when starting any new habit, and that includes beginning some kind of daily or thrice weekly breath work practice. Don't sabotage yourself by being too ambitious in the beginning. Set yourself a goal that you *know* you can achieve and be realistic about your time constraints and your motivation. It's better to say, "I'll do ten minutes each day" and do it throughout the week consistently than to attempt a daily one-hour practice that lasts through Tuesday and is abandoned as yet another failed health regimen. If you have had trouble in the past starting something new make an agreement to do only three movements or exercises. Once you've broken the ice you should find the exercises are absorbing and, what's more, you feel so good you want to go on. If you don't set up a high wall to climb over, you will be less likely to balk.

Studies have shown that people who exercise in the morning are more successful in establishing and maintaining their program over a period of time. Doing your practice in the morning sets the tone for the day. If you honestly can't stomach any activity in the morning, late afternoons before dinner are also an opportune time to come down from the activities of the day. I don't recommend practicing before bed (unless you are specifically working on relaxing to go to sleep), because most of these exercises will leave you wide awake.

At the end of this book, you'll also find Practice Guides for specific problems such as insomnia and asthma, as well as suggestions for retraining breath-holding patterns such as hyperventilation or reverse breathing. These programs help you to put all the information in this book into a logical sequence that you can use on a daily basis. There's also a "general" guide that outlines a progressive program for those of you who have no particular medical problems or ailments, but want to improve and refine your breathing and increase your energy levels.

As you do the exercises and inquiries practice as if you were a musician—

honing your skill in creating an even and smooth sound to your breathing, a calm and regular rhythm, and a uniform and effortless motion. As you play the instrument of your body, let your breathing become a melody that you would never tire of hearing.

Preliminary Cautions

If you have an underlying health condition that is worsened by deep breathing, you may want to consult your physician before proceeding. In all the exercises you should never strain or reach a point where you feel breathless. You might believe that it is only through working hard that you will make progress but it is just this sort of tension that will backfire, causing your brief efforts of "deep" breathing to be immediately followed by erratic, labored, and fast gasping. In particular you should *never* forcefully hold your breath. This is particularly important for people who have high blood pressure or a preexisting heart condition.

Don't do these practices directly after eating. Wait at least 2–3 hours after a heavy meal. You may also find that you need to drink more water after practicing breathing exercises as they can dehydrate the body.

Strengthening
Diaphragmatic Breathing

Note: A "cycle" of breathing consists of one inhalation and one exhalation.

You'll Need

2–3 blankets or a breathing bolster (see Resources)

> He lives most life whoever breathes most air.
>
> —ELIZABETH
> BARRETT BROWNING

Purpose

All breath holding patterns involve a partial contraction of the diaphragm. The following exercises loosen and strengthen this crucial muscle. If you haven't already acquainted yourself with the location and function of the diaphragm, take the time now to review the anatomy of your diaphragm in Illustrations 11 and 12.

Variation A

Recline in the Breathing Easy position (see Figure 32)or seated on a chair or cushion. Bring your hands down and wrap them around the base of your rib cage so that your thumbs are facing back and your fingers face toward each other (if you have a small rib cage your fingers may even touch each other) (Figure 33A). Press your thumbs firmly into the rib cage to create a slight resistance to the free movement of the ribs, but do not press your fingers into the soft depression underneath the tip of your breastbone. Now begin to direct and expand your breath into the ribs, expanding the ribs out to the sides against the pressure of your hands. Keep your eyes open in the beginning so you can see, as well as feel the movement of the diaphragm as it broadens. With each breath the fingers of the hands move away from one another and with each exhalation the hands come together, with the rib cage moving like an accordion.

Continue breathing in this way, providing firm resistance to the expansion of the rib cage so that your diaphragm and intercostal muscles must work to open. Check as you are breathing that you are not tightening the muscles in the upper chest, back, neck, or face. Rest after about 10 breath cycles, and allow your arms to come down by your sides as you let your breathing return to normal. Do another two sets of 10 cycles, resting for about 10 breath cycles between each set.

As you do the exercise, concentrate on creating a smooth and even movement rather than mechanically lifting the ribs up and down. Feel the ribs expand not only around the sides but throughout the back of the body as well. When

FIGURE 33A

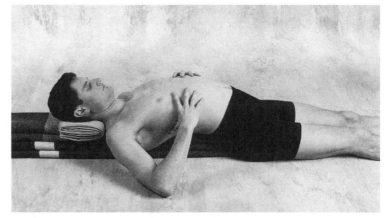

you are through with the three sets of ten, take a moment to check in with your breathing. How does it feel now? (If you wish, you can have a friend press her hands around your rib cage so you can focus on working the diaphragm while completely relaxing the arms and shoulder.)

Variation B: Sandbag Breathing

You'll Need

A 10-pound sandbag or a similar weight of beans or rice (see Resources)

Purpose

In this variation you use the weight of a sandbag instead of your hands to provide resistance to the diaphragm muscles. It's rather like weight lifting for your breathing muscles! The advantage of using the sandbag is that you can focus on relaxing your upper body and secondary respiratory muscles while you work the diaphragm. Although a 10-lb. sandbag might seem heavy, the weight is actually distributed over your middle so it feels more like someone pressing firmly on your body.

A sandbag is a very useful prop to have for strengthening the diaphragm. They take only 30 minutes to make, but you can also improvise by filling a plastic bag with beans or rice, or using a few of the rectangular bags of rice easily purchased at your local supermarket. Make sure, whatever you use, that it is about ⅓ empty so it wraps around your body rather than resting on you like a hard brick.

Here's How

Lie in the Effortless Rest position (see Figure 3, page 18) or completely supine on the floor with the legs extended. Now place the sandbag across the base of the ribs, directly underneath the breasts. It will cover the area from the middle ribs to the middle of the abdomen above the navel (Figure 33B). After you have taken a few moments to relax and check in with your breathing, begin to direct your breathing into the area underneath the sandbag. Rather than lifting the body with muscular effort against the sandbag, imagine that your body is having an easy conversation with the sandbag, gradually expanding and making contact all the way around the mid-torso. Concentrate your efforts for 10 breaths

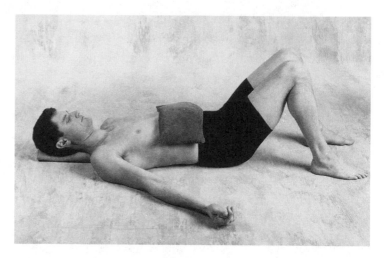

FIGURE 33B

and then rest, allowing your breath to breathe you without effort. Then repeat another two sets, resting in between each set. When you are through, take the sandbag off and observe your breathing. How are you breathing now?

Lengthening the Exhalation

~ INQUIRY ~

Straw Breathing[2]

You'll Need

A straw
A blanket, if you are reclining in the Breathing Easy position
A chair or cushion, if you are sitting

Purpose

Inhalation comes as a natural result of a full exhalation. In many breath holding patterns and most dramatically in lung disorders such as emphysema and asthma, the ability to exhale has been greatly diminished. The person may prematurely cut off the exhalation and then initiate their inhalation with the use of accessory respiratory muscles rather than using the diaphragm. Over time the habit of prematurely curtailing the exhalation can lead to more serious lung and heart problems.

When you breathe through a straw it takes longer to exhale. The beauty of this exercise is that you aren't thinking about manipulating your breathing at all which can cause mental tension and frustration—you are simply breathing through a long straw.

Here's How

Recline in the Breathing Easy position (see Figure 32) or sit on a cushion or chair. Before you begin straw breathing do a check-in with your breath and count how many breath cycles you take per minute. Once you've established this base line, place a long straw in your mouth and hold on to it gently with your hands. Don't try to hold it without the help of your hands, or you will unnecessarily contract your facial and jaw muscles. Breathe *in* through your nose and then breathe *out* through your mouth into the straw, working gently so as not to push the breath out (Figure 34). When you take your next breath in, lightly touch your tongue to the roof of your mouth to prevent yourself from breathing in through your mouth. Continue for 3 minutes. At the end of each exhalation concentrate your attention on allowing the inhalation to arise spontaneously. When the diaphragm initiates the inhalation it will feel like a gentle "bounce" up through the center of your body. If you can allow this to happen, the incoming breath will be effortless. We usually don't trust this to happen and jump in prematurely by initiating the inhalation with our upper chest and shoulders. Toward the end of your 3-minute session, count the number of breath cycles per minute again.

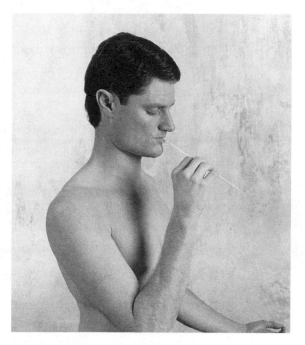

FIGURE 34

Has it changed? Over time you can increase your straw breathing sessions to 10–15 minutes.

A word of warning. Some people feel a sense of panic when they first try the straw experiment. I believe this is because increasing the length of the exhalation is "counter-intuitive"—that is, we're convinced we have to put the emphasis on the inhalation or we won't get enough air. If you feel uncomfortable, just stop and take a few normal breaths until you feel relaxed and calm again. I encourage you to persevere, as I did, because the results are truly dramatic. After doing this exercise I have noticed that both my inhalations and exhalations dramatically lengthen and the action of my diaphragm becomes smoother and more languid. Some students have reported feeling calm and relaxed for 3 to 4 hours after only 10 minutes of straw breathing. In group classes most students *halve* the number of breath cycles they take after only 5 minutes of straw breathing, without feeling any strain whatsoever. Because this is such a powerful exercise I try to incorporate it into my daily routine as a way of setting the metronome of my breathing for the day. You can do this breath work as a part of your sitting meditation, or as a quietening exercise before you go to bed. You might also carry a straw with you and take a few long exhalations before every meal.

The following are some other ways you can increase your exhalation using the same principles as the straw work. These variations may be helpful for children (particularly those with asthma) who might otherwise be unable to maintain the concentration needed for the previous exercise. These variations are also great for young-at-heart adults!

- **Blow through a musical instrument** Recorders and harmonicas are cheap and ideal for children.

- **Blow bubbles** into the air, or blow bubbles into water with a straw. See how long you can blow each stream of bubbles without straining.

- **Sing a song** Singing is nothing more than a melodious exhalation. If you are self-conscious, sing in the shower.

- **Chant** Chanting sacred verses and prayers is especially powerful because these songs are generally very rhythmic. There are many wonderful audio tapes that you can use to learn a variety of chants. Chanting Sanskrit (an ancient Indian language) is particularly powerful as the sounds of the words are designed to vibrate and balance the entire body. Continuous chanting for 5, 10, or even 20 minutes has a profound effect on breathing, as well as inducing a very peaceful state of mind.

- **Licorice Whips** Use a hollow licorice whip instead of a straw. This is a fun game to play with a child to help him or her calm down—or you can do your breath work surreptitiously on the bus or subway on the way to work. When you are through you can destroy the evidence by eating it.

～ INQUIRY ～

Sounding the Exhalation

You'll Need

Blankets, if you are lying down
Cushion or chair, if you are sitting

Purpose

Exhaling through pursed lips or by making sounds creates a resistance to the outgoing air, which maintains the intra-airway pressure. This prevents the premature collapse of the airways so that exhalation becomes easier.[3] Because air is being exhaled more slowly than it would be if you breathed out through an open mouth (try it so you can feel the difference) the body is tricked into making the exhalation longer. These deep exhalations cause a spontaneous increase in the depth of the subsequent inhalation.

Here's How

Sit or lie in the Effortless Rest position (see Figure 3). Take a full, easy inhalation through your nose. As you exhale, sound the syllables *wu, ee,* and *ah* on separate exhalations.[4] At first, sound each syllable for 5 to 6 seconds. Take a normal breath in and out between each syllable. Gradually increase the length of your sung exhalation until you are sounding for 15–20 seconds. It's important that you don't strain or you will resort to your old strategies of grabbing for the inhalation prematurely. After sounding the exhalations twice, return to normal breathing and see if your exhalation is fuller and longer. Notice whether you are breathing more fully into your diaphragm. If you have a preexisting condition such as asthma, take your time in increasing the length of time you exhale. You can build up to doing the sounds for 5–10 minutes in a session. Remember, never strain so that you feel short of breath. Your measure for success is a smooth, open, and easy feeling to your breathing.

～ INQUIRY ～

The Three-Part Breath

You'll Need

3–4 blankets, folded to make a 3-inch high, 8 by 10-inch wide, and 3 by 4–feet long bolster, or use a breathing bolster (see Resources)

Purpose

In this inquiry, you trick the body into lengthening the exhalation by dividing the exhalation into three parts, pausing briefly between each successive exhalation. The combination of the staggered exhalation and the pauses in between create a longer exhalation than you might normally take. This lengthened exhalation in turn stimulates a deepening of the inhalation. This is an especially helpful exercise to do if you have difficulty falling asleep. It is also an effective technique for diminishing anxiety that doesn't seem to have any particular source, and for those times when there is a buildup of tension in the body as often happens before the menses or during menopause.

Here's How

Assume the Breathing Easy position (see Figure 32) or lie in the Effortless Rest position (see Figure 3). Spend a few minutes to settle yourself and to consciously relax the body. To begin the exercise, take a normal breath in and then divide your exhalation into three equal parts, pausing very briefly between each part. It will sound something like this:

> Inhalation
> exhale-pause,
> exhale-pause,
> exhale-pause,
> Inhalation
> One or two normal breaths in and out, then repeat from beginning.

If you have a very weak respiratory capacity you may need to take more normal breaths in and out between cycles. Then begin again, inhaling, followed by a staggered exhalation, letting each part of the exhalation be the same length as the others. The pause should be a moment of suspension as when you say *ah*, rather than a feeling of contracting or holding the breath. If you feel short of breath you are probably trying to make the exhalations or the pauses too long. Adjust until you feel completely relaxed with no sense of grabbing for the inhalation. Also make sure that you are not breathing in or out during the pause.

You may find that images can help you create a smooth, even rhythm. I like to picture the breath movement as a waterfall flowing down, collecting in a pool during the pause, and then flowing down to the next pool. Or you can imagine that you are scaling down a tall ladder, exhaling as you step down, pausing at each step and then descending further. Some students like to envision that they are going down an elevator and stopping on each floor. It is most important that you don't strain, so feel free to go back to normal breathing, consciously relaxing and letting go of any striving or efforting. The less you try, the less you strive, the longer the exhalation will become. Continue with this exercise for a total of about 10 cycles of staggered exhalation and then completely relax. Take a few minutes to feel the effects of your practice before you continue with your day.

Stimulating the Breath

～ INQUIRY ～

Kapalabhati (The Cleansing Breath)

You'll Need

A cushion or chair to sit on
An empty stomach (wait 2–3 hours after eating before doing this practice)

Purpose

Known by some as the "breath of fire," *kapal* means "skull" and *bhati* means "to cleanse, light, or luster." I like to think of this yogic practice as a technique that makes the brain shine. Kapalabhati is a rapid exhalation breath pattern aided by strong abdominal contractions. Because kapalabhati quickly oxygenates the blood, one feels alert and revived after only a few minutes of practice. It can be used as a regular "wake-up" exercise or a "pick-me-up" practice whenever you feel down in the dumps or lethargic. It also helps tone your abdominal muscles. Further, carbon dioxide levels are decreased as stale air is expelled from the lower lungs, and the body is simultaneously saturated with oxygen.

In previous chapters I've warned against hyperventilation, which causes a lowering of blood carbon dioxide. Kapalabhati is different for two reasons. Most important, you *are consciously breathing this way to produce a certain effect,* and unlike hyperventilation you are exhaling completely and fully. In hyperventilation one tends to grab for the inhalation after an incomplete exhalation. In Kapalabhati the inhalation happens spontaneously. Nonetheless you should not do this practice forcefully or to excess so that you feel agitated and tense. Rather it should leave you feeling alert and glowing.

Some Cautions: This practice should not be done right after eating, nor during menstruation or pregnancy as the strong abdominal contractions would be harmful at these times. Those with heart complaints and high blood pressure should also avoid this practice, and people with herniated discs (commonly known as slipped discs) may find the strong abdominal pressure irritates their back problem.

Here's How

Begin by sitting on a cushion or chair with your spine relaxed and long. Take a few moments to check in with your breathing. Then begin to draw your lower abdomen inward on exhalations, while allowing the inhalation to arise spontaneously. Do this three or four times until you get the hang of the abdomen moving like a bellows. Now begin to speed your exhalations so that you take an exhalation every second. You'll sound a little like "the little engine that could" as you stroke with the abdomen. The exhalation is active and the inhalation should be completely passive. After a minute, rest and breathe normally for about 10 breaths before you begin another round of quick exhalations. Do three rounds in all, taking time to rest and breathe normally in between the rounds. When you become adept at breathing out every second, you can try breathing out every half second so that you take 120 exhalations per minute. Make sure that you are not tensing the upper body, eyes, or face but keep the action centered in the lower abdomen—stroking the breath in light brisk movements on each exhalation. Between each round simply watch how your breathing is changing. It may be deeper or longer than usual. Also observe how your mental state changes and whether you begin to feel more vibrant in your body.

Once you've become adept at doing Kapalabhati through both nostrils you can practice it through one nostril at a time. Do three rounds closing the left nostril and breathing in and out through the right nostril, making sure that you rest between rounds. Then switch to the left nostril for three rounds. Finally, finish your practice by breathing through both nostrils for two to three rounds.

Always take some time afterwards to feel the effects of the practice. Once you know how the practice affects you personally, you can decide when to use it. The next time you feel the urge for a caffeine pick-me-up try Kapalabhati instead.

Stimulating Your Breathing Through Exercise

One of the simplest ways that you can deepen your breathing is to do some activity that requires a slight physical exertion. It is not uncommon to go through an entire day without having done anything that actually required the body to breathe deeply. Cars, elevators, escalators, and other conveniences combined with sedentary occupations eliminate many opportunities, but here are a few suggestions:

Walk! Walk! and Walk! Whenever you have a chance walk up stairs instead of taking an escalator or elevator, walk up hills, or park your car a few blocks from work and take a brisk walk. Walk at a pace at which you feel your breathing quicken and deepen but never so that you are so puffed that you can't keep up a conversation. Walk in the clean and invigorating air as often as you can, especially if you are fortunate enough to live near a beach or woods. If you live in the city, try walking very early in the morning when the air is at its freshest.

Exercise doesn't need to be a compartmentalized activity. Walking is the most natural and the easiest to incorporate it into your life. My sister, who decided she wanted to be fitter, takes a daily walk up a long hill to the hospital where she works as a psychiatric nurse. After six months of this activity, her skin coloring, her vitality, and her energy level are noticeably different and she is back to her pre-pregnancy weight. Although she must get up an hour earlier to enjoy her walk (no small feat for a woman with two demanding children), she feels much more energetic. When you walk, try to get into a rhythm with your breathing rather than using the time to worry about unresolved problems.

Other exercises that are particularly good for eliciting deep breathing are bicycling (build from riding on flat land to to more challenging hills), and swimming (start with one length at a time followed by a rest period and work up to doing 10 lengths or more at one stretch).

If you do a particularly aerobic exercise such as running it's important not to fall back on old strategies such as chest breathing or hyperventilating. This can be especially true in aerobic fitness classes where people often resort to panting and chest breathing in order to keep up with the rest of the class. If you are not compelled by any of these options or dislike the competitive nature of many exercise regimens, you may want to find a hatha yoga class in your local area (see Resources for national directories). Yoga is a complete physical and mental conditioning in which breathing plays an intrinsic role in each movement. It is also a science that one can apply to all aspects of one's life. Find something that you enjoy, and whatever you choose to do, start off slowly, making sure that you maintain diaphragmatic breathing.

Balancing the Breath

～ INQUIRY ～

Alternate Nostril Breathing

You'll Need

A cushion or chair to sit on

Purpose

This exercise helps to balance the body and mind as well as soothe and calm the nerves, leaving you in a mentally alert but relaxed state. It is a terrific way to combat the jitters before a potentially stressful event. I have used it before going on stage, before examinations and public presentations, and also during times when my thinking was confused or uncentered. My students have used it to combat fear of flying or as a simple way to center themselves after a particularly frazzling day at work.

There are literally hundreds of patterns that can be practiced in alternate nostril breathing, but we will concentrate on a basic practice which nonetheless creates a profound effect. (For more detailed information on nostril dominance and the anatomy of the nose refer to page 62.)

If you tend to be congested, you may want to do a nasal wash before this exercise. Even if you are not congested, a nasal wash will open your nasal passages and refresh the mind. For instructions, refer to page 64. If you do not have access to a sink, blow your nose thoroughly before you begin.

Here's How

Sit cross-legged on a cushion or sit on a chair if you find this more comfortable. Using the left or the right hand (it's good to alternate hands each time you practice), fold the index and third finger inwards to touch the palm near the base of the thumb. Bring the thumb and the tip of the ring finger together to touch. Let the little finger rest gently against the side of the ring finger.

Bow your head slightly downwards, as if you were going to put a hood over your head. As you make the gesture of bowing your head slightly downwards, let your awareness curve back into itself, cultivating a self-reflective state. Bring your hand up, open the thumb and ring finger, and place the tip of the thumb on the side of one nostril and the tip of the ring finger on the other nostril (Figure 35). The cycle is as follows:

1. Close the left nostril and exhale completely through the right nostril.
2. Inhale through the right nostril.
3. Close the right nostril and exhale through the left nostril.
4. Inhale through the left nostril.
5. Close the left nostril and exhale through the right nostril. This completes one cycle. Continue for up to 20 cycles, finishing by exhaling through the right nostril.

As you proceed with the cycles be careful that your hand is not pulling the head off center. Also check that you are not slouching forward with your chest. Keep your breastbone upright. Open your eyes briefly every 4–5 cycles and check your body position before closing the eyes and continuing. Also, let your fingers be sensitive so that as you close a nostril you are not pressing so hard that the septum is being pushed off center. When you complete your practice always take a few moments to observe the effects of your practice. How would you describe your state of mind?

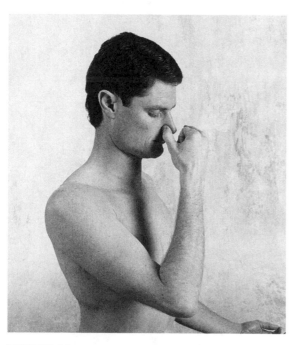

FIGURE 35

Alternate Nostril Breathing with Counting

Once you have become adept at the basic form of alternate nostril breathing you can begin to time each segment of the breath by mentally counting. In this way, the inhalation and exhalation will be exactly the same length. Start with a number that is absolutely comfortable such as four and gradually build up to six, eight, ten and even twelve counts for each phase of the breath. Do not increase the length of the count if you have even the slightest sensation of strain or discomfort. The lengthening of the breath cycle should arise as a result of opening and relaxing and not through force or aggressive use of your will power. Counting can be an excellent way of keeping the mind focused, especially if you have a tendency to drift off.

On page 199, you'll find Practice Guides, programs that will help you put all the information in this book into logical sequences that you can use on a daily basis.

VII

The Shared Breath:
Inquiries for Couples

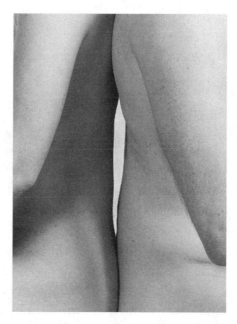

A man and a woman sit near each other;
as they breathe they feed someone we do not know,
someone we know of, whom we have never seen.

—ROBERT BLY

As we learn to listen to our breathing we develop greater skill in knowing who we are and what we feel at any given time. We can learn to use the breath as a Geiger counter to sense, locate, and define our experience. The clarity that this information provides allows us as individuals to reconcile what we feel and what we do. It helps us match our words and actions to our values and beliefs. And in relationships we can only communicate with precision if we know what our own feelings, needs, and desires are. This clarity allows us to be honest and loving with one another. Lacking this, our relationships can become a quagmire of confusion and misunderstanding.

To know what we are feeling and what is important to us, we must inhabit the body. We feel the body through the medium of the breath. In the previous inquiries you may have started to make correlations between sensations in your body and your emotional states. When you are angry, sad, afraid, or joyful, you feel certain sensations in your body. You open (or close off) to the information of these sensations by either allowing your breath to move through your body or by holding your breath. When you keep your breath moving you open a vast "body dictionary" of information that is infinitely more accurate and reliable than your ideas and preconceptions. When you are not sure about something you can check your perceptions in this internal body dictionary. For instance, you may be able to recognize how a combination of sensations, tensions, and breathing changes equals "I'm exhausted" or "I don't trust that person!" or "I feel confused." The more adept you get at comprehending these perceptions the easier it will be to place yourself on a solid ground and engage in an accurate and clear understanding—both with yourself and with others.

At times trusting and following our body-based perceptions can be difficult, as the messages we hear from our bodies may conflict with our preconceptions about the way our life should proceed. These body-based perceptions may also be in conflict with the ideas that other people have about what is right for us, from the job that we hold to whether we should have a child. The good news is that the body doesn't lie. The good bad news is that the onus now falls on you to listen and act from these body-based perceptions. The better you become at doing this for yourself, the more proficient you will become at knowing what you want and communicating that to your partner. You'll also become more skillful at reading your partner's body language.

The wonderful thing about working with body-based perceptions is that you are working with a palpable form. In a relationship one can often become entangled in an endless struggle to gauge and decipher feelings, emotions, and motives. It is far easier to work at the tangible level of the body than to alter emotions, attitudes, or intransigent opinions. When one opens the body to greater fluidity other aspects of the psyche follow suit.

In group classes I often have the opportunity to observe the way couples embody their "issues." As their somatic experience changes, the relationship inevitably undergoes dramatic changes. Chris and Patty began coming to yoga classes at the beginning of their relationship. What was most striking to me about Chris was his inability to relax his body during exhalation. He would breathe out but keep his muscles tense and rigid. As I got to know the couple I discovered Chris was a lawyer who worked long hours. He had a big, expensive home but had little time to enjoy it—an irony he was perceptive enough to recognize. He also seemed to be very reluctant to make any commitment to Patty, and would withhold expressing feelings for her. He was a forceful and opinionated person, which, I imagined, might not make him easy to be around. In short, he was a person for whom life was one long inhalation. One day, after trying a new breathing technique he finally understood what it meant to let his entire body exhale. Not long after this he confided that he was giving up his expensive home so he wouldn't have to work such long hours and he had decided to make a commitment to his relationship.

This chapter is about learning to use your breath as a way to connect with your own body-based wisdom. It is also about learning to connect with your partner in a more embodied way. Most of the inquiries that follow are designed to be done with a partner. Working with another person can help you to develop the very same quality of attention you need to give yourself. I have noticed in the seminars I lead that when people are partnered up to do an exercise they are more attentive than if they did the exercise by themselves. The beauty of a relationship is that as you learn to listen to another person, you are developing the skills to listen to yourself. As you notice changes in your own body movement and breathing quality you become more adept at distinguishing these things in others. You are then working together to heighten your sensory awareness in a way that will help create and sustain a healthy relationship.

~ INQUIRY ~

Mapping Body-Based Sensations

In the next week make special note of the body-based sensations you experience when you have particular feelings. When you notice yourself feeling a certain way, take a moment to breathe fully and to use your breath to locate and define your experience. In particular, notice the body-based sensations you experience when you are in dialogue with your partner. For instance, when I get angry at my partner I tend to contract into a frozen breathing pattern that acts as a fortress between myself and my partner. When I have the courage to soften and open my breathing, I notice that my partner is more willing to listen to me. How do you experience your breathing when there is conflict or ease between you? Are you comfortable enough to tell the truth to each other based on your somatic perceptions?

Fostering Intimacy: Touching from the Inner Body

When we touch each other in a relationship we often touch with our physical bodies but we do not touch each other from the feeling part of ourselves. It is not unusual for people to feel, even during the very intimate contact of sexual intercourse, that they remain untouched and disconnected from their lover. This superficial way of relating is hard to quantify in words, and no doubt has been the subject of endless futile and painful discussions that give neither partner much help. What can be quantified is the level at which we engage with one another physically and how that translates to a quality of intimacy or a sense of alienation. It is possible to touch only with your outer body, and here I mean quite literally your skin, muscle, and bone, and to withhold from your inner body—the soft organs, the blood, the circulating fluids, and the breath that moves through all of these substances. Although the idea of superficial and deep layers of the body corresponding to levels of connection may sound simplistic, I can assure you that working with the tangible body is far more likely to bring you and your partner a sense of deepening intimacy than endless discussions of subjective emotions. Take a moment to try the following simple exercise to experience for yourself just what I mean.

～ INQUIRY ～

The Inner Body Embrace

This is one of my favorite exercises to do with couples in a group. Once you've tried this it will leave no doubt in your mind about the quality of touch and connection that you would want from a loved one. Because we're talking about particular structures rather than nebulous ideas it also becomes much easier to communicate what you need from your partner.

Stand apart with your eyes closed and take a moment to feel the outer layer of your bodies: your skin, your muscles, and your bones. Feel how this outer layer gives you both containment and separation from everything in your environment. As you hug your partner, embrace him with these superficial layers. Feel your own body as well as the other person's body. Notice where you touch and where you don't. Feel the other person's skin, muscles, and skeleton. When you hug let only this external layer of yourself come into contact with your partner. It's quite likely that your bellies won't even touch and that you move your hips back, away from the other person. Also notice the quality of your breathing. Now stand apart and take a moment for your perceptions to come through.

Now sense into the soft inner organs in your body. Your beating heart, the lungs inflating and deflating, your stomach and your guts and your sex organs. Feel your breath moving through the soft contents in your body—expanding from the core to the skin. Now embrace your partner from these deeper structures. Feel the inner contents of your body making contact with your lover. Feel your breath making contact with her body. Notice how much more of your body makes contact with the other person (Illustration 32). Also see if you can feel where your partner yields to you, where you open and surrender to her, and where you hold back. Did this embrace feel more intimate or more satisfying? What did you feel your partner was communicating to you through her body?

The next time you hug someone notice how much of yourself you make accessible. How much do you soften your boundaries, and how much do people extend this openness to you? It is not always appropriate to give such intimate embraces, but by learning to distinguish the level at which you are engaging you will be more aware of appropriate boundaries for the given situation.

The Movement of Love

Love-making reduced to its basic components is the undulating breath. It is the ebb and flow of a primal wave movement. The source of this rhythm lies in the swelling and receding motions of the pelvis and the abdomen as they open to the incoming breath and draw inward on the outgoing breath. Allowing the root source of the breath in the lower body to move freely generates a wave that can travel both up and down the body. As this happens we also allow pleasurable, but not necessarily sexual, sensations to arise uninhibited. You may want to review the inquiries in chapter 2 that focus on the movement of the abdomen, pelvic floor, pelvis, and sacrum (also see Illustrations 1 and 2).

Just as breathing is a global body experience, love-making is a whole-bodied experience—a "polymorphous sensuous-

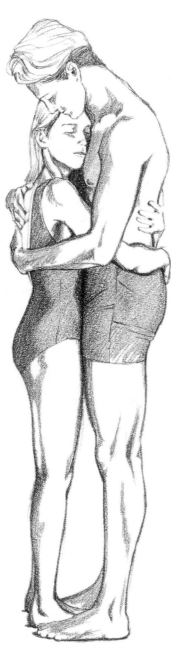

32. *Inner body embrace*

ness," as psychologist Michael Washburn describes in his book *The Ego and the Dynamic Ground,* in which the capacity for aliveness and pleasure permeates each and every cell of the body. In a culture as genitally fixated as ours, large expanses of the body are designated irrelevant territory and thus ignored. When this localized focus shifts to a more whole-bodied perspective, we can multiply by a hundred our capacity to love and be loved, to feel pleasure and to give pleasure, and to experience ourselves as a whole rather than a part.

Unfortunately, just as most of us have misconceptions about what it means to take "a deep breath" few of us arrive as adults without a bulging bag of ideas and concepts about what it means to love and what it means to have "great sex." Just as the strategies of effort, force, and willpower only sabotage full spontaneous breathing, these same ideas translate in the sexual arena to aggressive, exaggerated, and mechanical gestures that serve only to deaden the senses. Just as we are taught to breathe deeply in self-defeating and energetically wasteful ways, the caricaturist love-making styles modeled to us through advertising, books, and film inculcate their own message. "Good sex" in the mind of the collective culture translates to aggressively pneumatic, thrust till you bust, Harold Robbins robotic athletics. We are taught to strive in the sexual arena only to discover that while we can mimic we cannot derive meaning.

It is the predilection of our work-ethic culture to believe that we must make and manipulate all things in our lives, including the desire for and act of sex. We may feel compelled to live up to a routine of sexual activity that does not honor our deeper rhythms. This natural cycle, where sexual desire waxes and wanes like the cycle of the moon, allows us necessary periods of solitude, self-reflection, and regeneration, without which deep connection with another is impossible. When we impose the pressure of schedule and performance on ourselves we interfere with the natural generation of our inner desires and do not allow our-

> As soon as the fire and water come together, the whole lodge is filled with white, hot steam—Tunkashila's Breath. . . . Grandfather's White Breath unites us, makes us one. It fills every vein, every cell in our body, and every cranny of our little hut.
>
> That breath, that hot steam, is recycled. It might have been inhaled and exhaled by a dinosaur, a plant, a mouse, or a famous chief of yore. It might be the breath of a dead grandparent of yours. Because of this breath, those who have come into the lodge as enemies will leave as friends."
>
> —ARCHIE FIRE LAME DEER

selves the time and ease of letting the wave of desire develop on its own. In her book *Mindful Spontaneity* author Ruthy Alon describes the way effort can stifle rather than stimulate love-making:

> Both men and women recognize the paradox that directly investing more effort, more ambitious motions, and placing more demands on the sexually located movement does not guarantee greater arousal. Perhaps even to the contrary, this effort undermines it. If you express your desire to encourage Nature by making every possible effort, then the flowing wave doesn't have a chance to endure . . . with a mentality that believes in the most and the strongest, people are driven to use the language of ever-increasing force. At the critical moment, when their involuntary system doesn't support their sexual intentions, they deal with it by investing more physical effort, more tension, more rigidity; and here lies the trap. The greater the effort in all other parts of the body, the more blocked will be the fragile wave of sex . . . you think you are stepping on the gas, but actually you are hitting the brakes.[1]

The moment opens, in it are contained like tiny seeds a million more divisions.

—WILLIAM KOTZWINKLE

The inquiries that follow are designed to help you explore the ways you can use your breath to enhance feelings of intimacy, raise your pleasure levels, and improve communication in your relationship.

Before You Begin

These inquiries are simple things that you can do with your partner to increase your sensitivity to each other and to open into a greater sense of pleasure in each other's company. It is best not to enter into these inquiries with a specific expectation, such as getting sexually charged, because such an agenda will make it virtually impossible to open to the myriad other ways you can be together. For many of us, sexual interaction takes the form of a mechanical progression from A to B to C, with predictable signals leading to a rote conclusion. What might happen if we didn't know where A led to? What might happen if instead of relating on this mechanical level we let ourselves embrace each moment with no set agenda? What if, as we pause and feel our breathing soften, we followed the natural flow and let ourselves melt into sleep together instead of feeling pressured to perform our predetermined ritual? Or might it lead us into a very quiet and deep sexual connection that allows us to regenerate, or into a wildness that we had not experienced before? The less investment you have in a specific outcome the more you can engage with one another in a new and renewing way.

It is quite possible that sexual sensations may arise spontaneously during some of these inquiries, and they are to be neither encouraged or discouraged. You may want to have an agreement with your partner before you do the inquiries as to what feels safe and comfortable for both of you. Read through this chapter and put an asterisk on inquiries that you'd like to try with your partner, and have him do the same. Then make your surroundings special in some way—flowers in the room, a candle burning, the room freshly cleaned and tidy. You may feel silly at first giving such conscious attention to things that you may already do casually, but it is the quality of your attention that can bring about the alchemy of transformation between you.

~ INQUIRY ~

The Shared Breath:
Back to Back Breathing

Sit back to back with your partner. Raise your buttocks with a cushion or pillow until your knees are slightly lower than your hips. Take a few moments to find a position in which you feel supported by your partner's back rather than feeling that your partner is pushing you forward. Begin by sensing your own breath, noticing your breathing pattern and rhythm. Then gradually shift your awareness to your partner's breathing. Slowly begin to synchronize your breathing so that you are breathing with your partner. This will take the full concentration of both people. Each of you will be making compromises and shifting your own breathing patterns to create a "shared" breath. As you breathe, open into the warmth of your partner's back against yours and the pleasure of breathing in unison. After about 5 minutes go back to breathing in your own rhythm. Now turn around and face each other with your knees almost touching. Take a moment to look each other in the eyes and to notice your unique breathing rhythm.

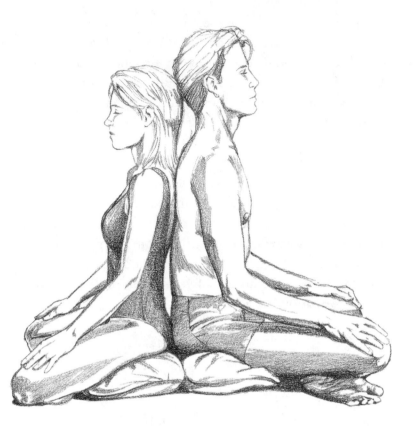

33. *Back to back breathing*

～ INQUIRY ～

The Gift of Presence

When we hurt, whether physically or emotionally, we want the kind presence of another to bear witness. We do not want explanations, advice, or trite platitudes, but a loving, compassionate attention. This attention lets us know that we are accepted even when we are not feeling bright and positive. Bearing witness to our own pain or providing a loving presence for another serves as an ongoing lesson that as human beings we come as a package of strengths and weaknesses, of positive and negative attributes.

This is an exercise that I often do to relax at the end of a class. After a few minutes of resting in a supine position I ask every person to scan their bodies and

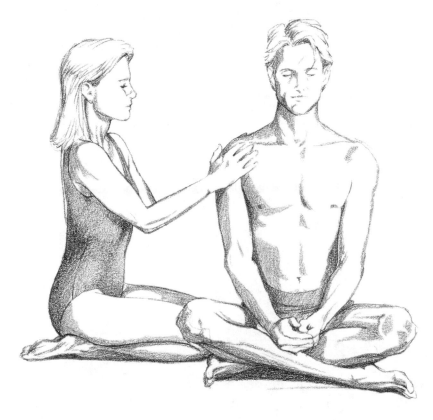

34. *The gift of presence*

find a place that refuses to relax. Everyone has these persistent spots of tension and holding that resist stretching, massage, and all other strategies. These are places where we don't breathe and where we store our greatest hurts and fears. Because of this we need to treat them with compassion and respect. After you and your partner have relaxed for a few minutes sit up and tell each other where you feel the most tension in your body. It might be a spot on your back, a sore hip or knee, or an ache behind your eyes. The next part is simple. You should now lie down again or sit in any position that is most comfortable. Your partner should simply place her hands on and around the area where you feel pain and tension. Her hands should be still and simply act as a presence (Illustration 34). It is not necessary to massage or manipulate. With her hands resting lightly on you, let your breathing move gently into the area. And ask yourself this question: Is there anything that I can *stop doing* in order to feel more breath flow into this part of me? See how much you can disengage from the action of holding. Feel your skin soften and the muscles loosen their grip on your bones. Feel your blood begin to circulate freely into the area of tension. The helping partner should begin to synchronize her breathing with yours, consciously exhaling more deeply and sensing for any changes in the tissue underneath her hands. Take 5–10 minutes each.

Many people are amazed at how such a seemingly passive exercise can allow them to release so deeply. The key is allowing your partner's help to bring your awareness to this blocked place within you. Frequently, when we feel pain in our bodies we have a truncated consciousness that does not travel into or through that part. Notice how it feels to have your partner's loving presence with you as you enter this vulnerable area. Take a few moments to share your perceptions and then switch roles.

～ INQUIRY ～

Speaking with "Breath Words"

Cuddling up against each other belly to back must be one of the all-time favorite pleasures for couples. "Spooning" can be done clothed or unclothed lying in bed or on any soft surface. Lie on your sides with one person curling around the other person's back. Make sure you both have pillows to support your necks. Now sense into the parts of your body that are in contact with your partner. Imagine that you are speaking to your partner with your breath—an intimate conversation that tells him how much you love and care about him. Feel these "breath words" arising from deep within your body and be receptive to hearing the breath words of your partner. Notice what sensations, images, and feelings arise. Allow yourself to move very slowly and gently as the urge takes you, but keep all movement small and smooth. As you relax your outer muscles do you notice more of your breath penetrating through to your skin and "speaking" to your partner? Be completely present with each other and the movement of each breath cycle.

You may want to stay in this position for 10–30 minutes, changing around as you feel the desire. If you are practicing the exercise in the evening, let yourself shift into a comfortable position and drift off to sleep together. If you are exploring the inquiry during the day, how much of this intimate communication can you maintain with each other throughout your daily interactions?

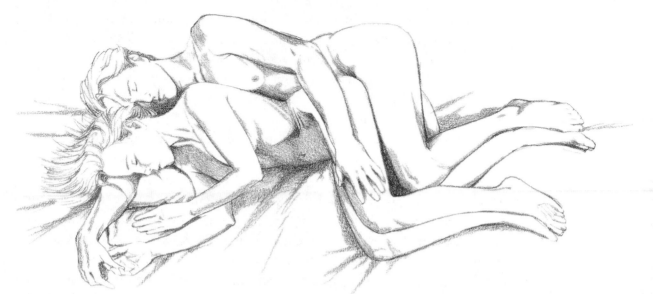

35 *Speaking with breath words*

~ INQUIRY ~

Belly to Belly Breathing

This inquiry can be done in many different ways and at different levels of intimacy. You can do the exercise completely clothed or naked, lying belly to belly on your sides, or with one partner lying on top of the other, and you can also do this exercise during sexual intercourse. Choose an option that feels comfortable to you. Although you may decide to explore this exercise during sexual intercourse its purpose is not necessarily to become sexually charged or to reach an orgasmic level of excitation. This may happen spontaneously, but you should not feel any pressure to produce a certain result or arrive at a predetermined conclusion. My partner and I often work with this inquiry and find that it works very nicely as a way to promote a very casual afternoon lie down, or to connect after we've been apart for weeks. When we explore the inquiry during sexual intercourse it doesn't always lead us to a highly charged state. However, since we do not have such expectations there is no disappointment if it doesn't happen; in fact, we often find the deep pleasure of quietly being with each other nourishes and replenishes us in a way that strenuous love-making sometimes does not. Listen and respond to each moment as it arises without prejudice and you may be pleasantly surprised. Just as close friends can allow for spaces of comfortable silence in their conversation, your ability to remain present with one another without feeling the need to do anything may be a gauge of how intimate you truly are with one another.

Lie with each other belly to belly, embracing and finding a position that feels comfortable for both of you. You may want to make eye contact, or you can close your eyes. Once again allow your breathing to arise from the deep core of your belly. Feel it spread throughout your abdomen, into your genitals, down into the fullness of your buttocks, and even into your thighs and legs. Allow the breath to dilate into your chest and back throughout your body so that you feel the entire body move slightly with each breath. Then begin to tune into your partner's body. It is not necessary to synchronize your breathing although this may happen spontaneously. Simply feel each other breathing and the expansion and contraction arising and subsiding as you breathe. If you are inside each other, be still with your body rather than thrusting or rocking. Simply feel your breathing. Notice the swell of the breath as it touches your body and allow whatever sensations and feelings that come on that tide to arise without suppression. Remember, you don't have to do anything with these sensations. You don't have to act on them. I often find that the longer I stay with my partner in this way the closer and more intimate I feel with him. Sometimes, without making any large movements or specifically orienting our attention genitally, the sheer act of breathing together can build a powerful sexual charge, as if a light were growing brighter and brighter. Again, this is not your goal, but if it happens spontaneously, do certainly enjoy it! By remaining still and continuing to breathe together you may be building a level of intimacy and pleasure that goes far beyond the pneumatic and mechanical sex that so many of us have experienced. Take as much time as you need to conclude the exploration. And remember that resolution doesn't necessarily mean having a mind-shattering orgasm. Each time you engage in this inquiry it may take you to a different place. The less you project your expectations the more potential there will be for something new to happen.

~ INQUIRY ~

The Wave of Breath

This last inquiry is for those of you who would like to explore the wave of breath during sexual intercourse. Choose a position that is comfortable for both of you and be open to changing positions at each other's request. As you enter each other, take a moment to pause in great stillness and rest. Feel each other and allow yourself to relax completely. Enter completely and be entered. As you rest in this moment of potential, feel the oscillation of your breaths and the subtle movement of the breath as your waves meet and rebound through each other's body. Instead of making large, impressive, or ambitious movements, allow yourself to remain receptive, feeling the presence of the other and your own internal sensations. Notice if you find it difficult to trust the process of allowing your sexual energy and connection to build of its own accord without "making it happen," and without manipulating each other's energy. Notice if you feel fear at this moment. Are you worried that you won't have an orgasm? Are you concerned that this sexual energy will dissipate or disappear if you cease to strive with effort?

As you remain in this position let your breath deepen throughout your belly. Spontaneously follow any impulse to move, letting yourself embrace, stroke, and enfold one another. Over time, a wave or charge may begin to form. If this does not happen it is not a sign of failure. You can continue to enjoy the pleasure of being with your partner. It can often take many sessions together before a charge will build. As you feel this, let this wave carry you, making very small, slow movements. As you begin to move slowly within and inside each other, notice how the smaller you make the movements the more you can feel. As you slow down you can feel the magnitude and power of each other.

Whenever you feel like pausing and remaining still, follow your instincts and allow yourself to be suspended in the feeling. These periods of stillness may last a minute or an hour. Let yourself swoon inside the buoyancy of those quiet moments. Let your love-making be an epiphany to the breath, honoring all phases

> The seeds stir and tremble
> as if the sky moves back and forth
> between us, like this, like this
> —SHARON GLADDEN

of the breath—the entering, the leaving, and the spacious pauses in between. Let this energy take you wherever it will, finding its own conclusion and resolution. When you have reached a resting place take some time with your partner to share your perceptions, listening to each other with your full attention. Are there elements of this love-making exercise that you might incorporate into other aspects of your relationship?

Knowing oneself and knowing another are two sides of the same coin. Just as the glaze on a piece of unfired pottery does not shine until fired, it is through the intense kiln of relationship that we come to be transformed. Many of our most deeply held fears, insecurities, and negative emotions will only arise and be resolved in the close quarters of a relationship. And many of our most intensely joyful experiences may only come through the alchemy of a relationship. With two psyches, two histories, and two perspectives, a relationship can become infinitely complex and potentially confusing. For this reason, it is crucial that each of you have a self-reflective practice where you can witness your own habit patterns, feelings, and sensations. This may take the form of a daily walk, a formal meditation session, or a nightly journal writing ritual, but it can also be a moment to moment conscious awareness of the breath. Each breath enters us, becomes a part of us for a moment and then is cast back into the world. For that moment we have a chance to know both who we are as an individual and who we are as the integral part of a greater shared breath.

VIII

Minding the Breath

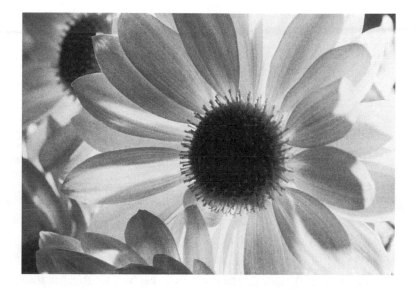

Enough. These few words are enough.
If not these words, this breath.
If not this breath, this sitting here.

This opening to the life
we have refused
again and again
until now.

Until now.

—DAVID WHYTE

Cultivating Mindfulness

To mind the breath is to make a decision. It may be the most radical decision you have ever made in your life. The second you choose to mind your breath you have decided that this present moment, this very moment, is worthy of your full attention. The instant you do this you have begun to extricate yourself from the hold of the past and the pull of the future. You are living your life as a today rather than a yesterday or a tomorrow.

> The man who sat on the ground in his tipi meditating on life and its meaning, accepting the kinship of all creatures and acknowledging unity with the universe of things, was infusing into his being the true essence of civilization.
>
> —LUTHER STANDING BEAR

What does it mean to be mindful and to cultivate mindfulness? It is simply that we notice the thoughts, feelings, and sensations that arise within us from breath to breath. We become aware of our breathing, our body, and our mind, and through this awareness come to peace with ourselves. Mindfulness means doing one thing at a time. We put our full attention on what we are doing, whether that be washing the dishes or driving the car, so we can be awake in that moment. After all, this moment will soon pass, and by being somewhere else we may not have lived it. All of life can pass in this way, each moment stolen by another that has not yet happened.

This awareness we are attempting to cultivate, by necessity, must be choiceless. It means that we stop deflecting, correcting, and manipulating our perceptions to suit our conceptual ideas about how we think we should be and how we think other people should be. It also means we open ourselves to the way our life is rather than how we imagine it should be. Of course, this is not the predilection of human beings. We're sure life should be a certain way and when it inevitably doesn't turn out as we had carefully planned we feel righteous anger or justifiable disappointment. Choicelessness is an extremely important principle to understand because mindfulness is not about reaching an idealized state of mind. The ultimate goal of mindfulness practice is not to attain a fairy-tale composure of sweetness where negative thoughts cease to exist. If you were to sit for even five minutes and watch the parade of jumbled and negative thoughts that dance on the screen of your mind (judgment, anger, and jealousy being likely contenders), you would realize in short order that such a goal is rather unrealistic. Neither should choicelessness be confused with blind or passive acquiescence to unacceptable or unhealthy situations or behaviors. It does mean that we see things as they are instead of embracing or dismissing our perceptions, holding on to things we like, or rejecting the things we dislike. In seeing things more clearly we can liberate ourselves from the endless roller coaster created by the opposing actions of attraction and rejection.

The other reason I emphasize the importance of entering mindfulness practice with choiceless awareness is that the very moment you strive for an ideal ego state which you call "good" you have simultaneously rejected another part of yourself which you call "bad." This rejected part of you doesn't just disappear; if unattended it may exist autonomously, unconsciously driving your behavior so that you make the same mistakes over and over again. It is thus best to place the shadow squarely before you where you can attend to it while doing your mindfulness practice rather than attempting to outrun it as it lurks behind you. You need not attempt to stop your thoughts; you need only change your relationship to your thoughts, feelings, and sensations. In the very act of looking clearly and unflinchingly at your feelings, however unsavory they may seem to you, you can begin to understand their root. If you relinquish embracing or dismissing you allow life to do what it has always done—to change.

Meditation is often associated with a struggle to attain some rarefied atmosphere of holiness and detachment in which one renounces all the things one enjoys. Ironically, the person who is not mindful of the present moment is in every breath renouncing true pleasure and delight. When we live outside the present we miss out on infinite opportunities to appreciate and enjoy the simple things that we do have. A cool glass of water on a hot day or the meal lovingly prepared goes unnoticed as we dwell on the possibility of more exciting moments.

Inquiring students often ask me whether meditation is merely an escape from the world, a running away from life. Far from escaping from "reality," mindfulness practice is one of the most radically confrontative practices one could choose. Rather than escaping from our fears, aversions, desires, and habits and retreating into some heavenly vacation resort for the mind, any true mindfulness practice forces us to see our negative thought patterns as well as to appreciate all the wonderful things about ourselves and others that we may habitually overlook.

Being mindful doesn't mean that we stop making plans or setting goals for the future. Awareness of this moment doesn't preclude learning from the mistakes of our past, or taking measures for the security of ourselves and our families in later years. But when we pay attention to the information we receive in the present we have a better chance of knowing where next to plant our feet. Listening to the clues and cues that come to us daily, our choices begin to reflect the fluid nature of life, so that regardless of our responsibilities and our schedules, there is always the possibility of making changes. Instead of working from rigid assumptions based on our experience or on our fantasy, we start to take our bearings from the "reality" of the present.

In the everyday hubbub and commotion of our lives it is indeed difficult to find this presence of mind. In the same way that you would not choose a racehorse as your mount for a first riding lesson, the turbulent chaos of daily activity may not be the best starting point for learning the skill of mindfulness. It is ultimately the ground where you must apply it, but in the beginning it is best to learn in the hothouse conditions of a formal practice. Creating ideal conditions for even 10 or 15 minutes will be rewarded tenfold in the quality of the rest of your day. "Ideal" means that you have a quiet place where you will be undisturbed so that you can listen to yourself without any added stimulation or challenges. Here are some suggestions for creating this space:

- Find or create a place, even if it is the corner of your bedroom, that is clean and uncluttered where you can sit or lie down. Make it special by lighting a candle, burning a stick of incense, or placing some fresh flowers in a bud vase. Over time this place will gain a certain power so that when you go there it will be easier to concentrate.

- Schedule an appointment with yourself each day, preferably at the same time. It need only be 10 or 15 minutes, but you must take it seriously. Others will inevitably try to get you to break this appointment. Don't.

- The quiet of early morning is very conducive to mindfulness practice. Set the alarm to wake you 30 minutes earlier. The energy you will have from your mindfulness practice will more than compensate for any lack of sleep.

- When you do your practice let others know that you are unavailable for that time. Close the door, turn off the radio, TV, and any music. Turn off the sound on the phone and let your answering machine do its job for a while. If you have no quiet space at home, consider doing your practice in a nearby park or library.

~ INQUIRY ~

Mindfulness Practice

(10–45 minutes: Gradually build up the time as your concentration improves.)

~ ~ ~

Sit in any position that you find comfortable. Lying down is not usually a good idea as your level of attentiveness is much diminished when you are supine. Close your eyes and let the weight of your buttocks settle into the cushion or chair. Notice if you are leaning forward anticipating the next moment, or if you are leaning back reclining into the past. Center the weight on your sitting bones so that you organize yourself to be present in the moment. Allow the contents of your belly to relax and begin to bring your awareness to your breathing.

It is this simple. Notice your breathing coming and going. Notice when the breath enters you and when it leaves you. Also pay attention to the pauses between the inhalation and the exhalation. As you sense and feel your breathing, thoughts, feelings, and sensations inevitably will arise. This mental activity is not a sign of failure. Note the feelings and sensations that arise in your body and heart. Detect sadness, excitement, or boredom. Be aware of the sensations arising in your body. You may feel certain areas becoming tense or heavy, you may notice your stomach gurgle or your heart beating. Simply note all of this without analyzing, judging, correcting, or solving. As you sit, an endless parade of thoughts, feelings, sensations arise and dissolve. They arise and dissipate without your effort. Imagine that you are like the sky and all these thoughts, sensations, and feelings are like clouds drifting by. Some stay for a while, some drift swiftly by, but they constantly change form. Amid all this fluctuation your breath is coming and going. Return your awareness over and over again to the breath, remembering that you are the sky, not the clouds of passing sensation. Do not become upset or reprimand yourself if you become captivated by a thought, feeling, or sensation and suddenly find that you have spent 5 minutes in a Joycean ramble. The important thing is that you notice what you are doing. The person who notices that he has drifted off and the person who is unconscious of his confusion are a thousand miles apart.

Can you let your breathing be just what it is? Without making it bigger, better, or different can you simply let the breath breathe you? How much can you disengage from effort and let the breath enter and leave on its own accord? Don't get caught up in a struggle with your mind. All thoughts, feelings, and sensations change. Simply allow yourself to be a sky for these drifting thoughts, returning over and over again to the steady rhythm of your breathing.

Each day as you do your mindfulness practice, notice what you have brought with you to your practice. Is it excitement, nervousness, anger, resentment, sadness, boredom, anticipation, fatigue? Simply noticing how you are brings a certain clarity to the day. You need not deflect or correct these constantly changing aspects of yourself. Simply be with yourself in this compassionate way, accepting who you are and how you are. When you finish your practice you may want to put your hands together in a gesture of prayer and bow forward, giving thanks for this day of living and breathing.

Breathing is a perfect tether for mindfulness practice because it is an ever-present reference point to which we can return again and again. When we breathe we are saying, "I accept what life brings me now." When we breathe into pain, we are saying we accept our pain. When we breathe into the experience of intimacy, we allow ourselves to absorb love and nourishment. When we hold our breaths or distort our breathing unconsciously, we attempt to barricade ourselves from life's trials. In doing so we miss life's treasures.

Being mindful isn't terribly easy because there is little support in our Western culture for such an awareness. We may feel that forces beyond our control transpire against us at every turn to erode our inner equilibrium. We say we feel "stressed out," frazzled, and overwhelmed. It will be helpful before we continue with other mindful breathing practices, to look at some of the obstacles that we may face.

Myths That Take Our Breath Away

The deeper causes of breath holding patterns must necessarily take us beyond discussions of stress and our reaction to it, and bring us face to face with our own confusion about our values, our accelerated lifestyle, and the cultural and social forces that may be holding us hostage. For some of us this will involve an archeological dig as we examine our personal history and the ways in which we recapitulate the traumas of the past and how this dictates the future. What is our

> It is far more difficult to murder a phantom than a reality.
> —VIRGINIA WOOLF

relationship to these forces? What we can know is that as long as we are held captive by unexamined phantoms, we will squander our life energy on pursuits and goals that bring us little real satisfaction. At the end of our lives we may stand baffled that we have strived so hard and for so long for things we never wanted in the first place.

Some myths lie so deep in the psyche that it is difficult to recognize their power over us. Traditionally myths were meant to act as clues to help us recognize what is important in our lives. Most of the modern myths, however, have led us not toward but away from finding the right relationship with ourselves and with others. The most significant of all these present-day myths is that of the successful person. When we are in the grip of this myth we are driven by the certainty that there must be a better moment than the one we find ourselves in. We have good reasons to be holding our breath—we've discovered we're living in the wrong moment! In this myth we are taught that we must aggressively compete, ends justifying the means, to "become someone" in order to "get there." "There" or what we will have when we reach this special place is never quite

> Most successful people are unhappy. That's why they are successes—they have to reassure themselves about themselves by achieving something that the world will notice . . . The happy people are failures because they are on such good terms with themselves that they don't give a damn.
>
> —AGATHA CHRISTIE

explained, but it is most certainly a place cluttered with beautiful things. Reaching this nirvana is all the justification we need for madly rushing about our lives, hyperventilating our way from one end of the day to the other. We dare not pause to take a breath and reflect lest we be left behind and miss out on the great reward. Curiously this reward seems to always be in the illusive future just out of our reach. "There," as it turns out, is a mirage.

On a recent airplane flight I used one of my frequent flyer coupons to travel first class. Next to me sat a very obese businessman who immediately struck up an animated conversation with me. He was beyond retirement age but not only chose to continue working eighty-hour weeks, he lived from Monday to Friday in a different state than his family, flying home only on weekends. He never missed a chance to make references that would let me know just how much money he earned: vacations in Italy, private schools for the children, a gorgeous home . . . but as the plane was making its descent he made a most remarkable statement. He told me that he had over five million dollars in stock and that "my wife and I think that we are almost 'there'; we're almost at the place we want to be." Then he turned to me and asked me about my work and I said that although, relative to his life standards, I didn't earn much money, I was able to decide how I would spend each day and each week so that I could enjoy my walks by the sea, my pleasure in cooking and gardening, and my beloved horse riding. "You know," he said pointedly, "I guess most of us are working so that we can do that one day!"

Sadly, that day never seems to come. More to the point, we may be so caught up in reaching this point that we find ourselves skipping over vast passages of our life as if we were speed reading. In the meantime, life goes on without us. We rush through the day, speeding up our seemingly menial tasks with machines and mechanization. It is almost as if we are under a mass hallucination, believing that time is running out. Indeed the myth that time is a vanishing commodity appears to both precede and follow the myth of the successful person. Not enough time to be civilized to each other, not enough time to extend a common courtesy, not enough time to stop for a pedestrian or to listen to the story of an elderly neighbor. You can help break the stronghold of this mass hallucination by extending time generosity to yourself and to others. The most fundamental way that you can do this is to take the time to breathe and do tasks "in your own time." Hurry-up sickness seems to be epidemic these days, and none of us is immune. Being mindful of your breathing is one of the best ways that you can avoid falling under the spell of the hurry-up hysteria.

You can also make choices that make hurrying less inevitable. For instance for many years I chose to bike as my form of transport. I was quite content getting about on my bicycle, by foot, or when necessary by bus. At the end of my first year of cycling to work, over five people at my workplace had bought bicycles and had joined me in my daily commute, so amazed were they at my growing fitness and exuberance. Ambrosia, my two-wheeled steed, slowed me down. She made it impossible for me to do too much in one day.

You can also take preventative measures against the hurry-up bug by taking time out to smell the roses. Late in her life, writer Alix Kates Shulman left the city to spend her summers in a primitive cabin in Maine. She returned there every summer for ten years reveling in uninterrupted days and profound solitude. Here is one of the things she discovered:

> Now time has stepped out of its running shoes, dropped its disguises, returned to the rhythm of the tides, the cycles of the planets and the moon, the slow ripening of the plants I gather, the long leavening of the yeasty breads I bake. Pointless to try to slow or hurry it, much less to "save" it. Slowly the kneaded dough rises in the bowl at its own pace, and after the first long rising you punch it down and let it rise again, and when it once more fills the pan, you bake it. The rich aroma of freshly baked bread permeates the cabin all day long, and each time you cut a slice, spread it with jam, chew it, you experience again the whole sensuous process: the kneading, the rising, the punching down, the baking. Gradually I realize that the very concept *saving time* is either a solecism (surely time goes at its own good pace) or a waste (save it for what?); the more lavishly I spend time, the more I seem to have, like the wild leaves I pluck for salad which grow more lushly the more I pick. In nubble time history melts away, taking with it all traces of the number game. *Old, young, obsolete*—these time-bounded words don't apply in a realm where there's time enough for everything; indeed, all the time in the world.[1]

～ INQUIRY ～

Extending Time Generosity

Each day give the gift of time to another. Imagine that you are passing on the good news that there's plenty of time for everyone. I like to become conscious of my breathing whenever I give a gift of time. Here are some of my favorites:

- In the check-out line at the supermarket let someone else with fewer things go before you. Tell them, "Please go ahead of me, I have plenty of time." Also, if you notice the cashier rushing to tally your goods, say, "Don't rush on my account, I'm not in a hurry. Take your time." And by the way, see if you can wait until the customer before you has put away his wallet before you step up to the cashier counter.

- Stop when you notice a pedestrian about to cross the road. Wait until they are all the way across instead of nudging the person along. Also, when you are crossing the street, walk at a pace that feels good to you rather than letting drivers intimidate you into trotting out of their way. Remember it's their hurry, not yours! Just make sure you don't challenge their steel contraption with your flesh and blood!

- Is there a task that you usually consider "menial" that you normally speed up? There are countless ways that we do this, from buying frozen spinach instead of the fresh that needs to be carefully washed, to driving to the corner market instead of taking the time to walk. At least once a day do one task that you usually speed up, by hand and without acceleration.

- Observe this week how many times you hold your breath "in order to (fill in the blank)." Phrases like "when I finish this report, then I'll relax" and "once I've finished the laundry, I'll relax" are clues as to how you may be constantly holding the present moment hostage for an imagined future. All of these skipped moments sometimes add up to a lifetime.

～ INQUIRY ～

The "Just This" Meditation

Whenever you feel yourself falling under the spell of busyness, try this simple meditation. You can do it anywhere and practice it for as long as 30 minutes or as briefly as one breath cycle. It is particularly effective when done while walking very slowly. Each time you plant your foot to step forward mentally say "just," and as you shift your weight onto your foot say "this." Or you can use your breath as a guide: each time you inhale say "just" and each time you exhale say "this." As you mentally steady yourself, take in just what's happening at that moment; not all the things you have left to do, or all the problems that have not yet been solved, but just your breath or your footstep planted on the ground. No matter how difficult or insurmountable a situation appears in its entirety, there are few things that cannot be managed when handled one increment at a time.

The History of Your Breath

We learn how to breathe in the milieu of family and friends. What has happened to us in the past can imprint itself on the way in which we breathe today. Trauma, fears, and chronic insecurities in our pasts can become cellularly encoded so that regardless of our chronological age we may continue to be a child for the rest of our lives—living and breathing as if every day were a series of yesterdays.

While few people can stake claim to having had a perfect childhood, there are many whose formative years left such deep scars that those wounds continue to cast a dark shadow on all of life's present pursuits. Knowing how we were wounded can help us to understand ourselves and our reactions better. This knowledge can also help us avoid stepping in the same puddles over and over again. When we open to our breathing we open ourselves to the knowledge of our personal wounds, but in doing so we also open ourselves to information that can help us to move beyond them.

As a child I lived in fear of moving to new places. We moved to new towns and countries often, and having no control over when I would be uprooted, I found the constant readjustment to new places and new people very distressing.

Eric spent many years living as a monk in a Zen monastery. In his first year he underwent a tremendously painful and emotional time. Completely overwhelmed by the intensity of his feelings he sought out the guidance of the head abbot. As he sat before the abbot he explained his dilemma and with great hope waited for the abbot to advise him as to how he might alleviate his suffering. The abbot answered simply "If you can breathe in . . . you can breathe out."

After a while I started to draw my shoulders together and hold my arms tightly clamped to my sides, hoping that this would make me less conspicuous to other children in each new school I attended. I began to breathe very shallowly and because I was rejected by other children and frightened of their taunts, I also began to breathe as if cringing from the cold. I was always on the alert for a leg that would trip me up in a hallway, or an object thrown at the back of my head in class. One professor specializing in breathing disorders described me recently as "intrinsically vigilant." To this day you can see the history of that childhood in the way I organize my body, although now I am aware of it, working to open and release these vulnerable places within myself. It has taken some time to change my breathing patterns and my body posture to inhabit my present life and leave my history behind me. Even today, I am aware of my tendency in certain situations to fall back into old ways of coping, like a rubberband springing back to its original size. Thankfully, as my breathing opens, these episodes are few and far between.

We become a certain person when we breathe in a certain way. You may want to examine your own personal history and look at the ways it has shaped the way you are today.

～　～　～

During your mindfulness practice notice any feelings that arise. Especially be aware of emotions that seem particularly strong and repetitive. Instead of deflecting these feelings or expressing them in action, simply take them in with each breath. Notice how your breathing changes as your feelings change. There's no need to hold on to a feeling or to analyze it, but if it does persist, let your presence keep it company. As you stay open with your breathing and being, the feeling will ripen and become more concentrated so that you experience the "essence" of the emotion. At other times you may discover that there is something else generating the feeling. In this way you can come to know some of the forces that drive your behavior.

All breathtaking myths have one thing in common. They are so powerful and so prevalent in all areas of our society that we rarely question them. Usually it is not until we meet a serious life crisis that we are forced to look at the way these unconscious forces drive our lives. Although pain continues to be a primary motivator for change in human beings, we need not wait for a crisis to decide we want to live differently.

Any activity that promotes self-reflective consciousness has the potential to be life changing. Taking the time to breathe and to absorb and assess what is important to you is one of the most politically and socially powerful actions you can take in your life. What might happen if you developed a clear perception of your feelings, emotions, and intuitions? If you had a sharper understanding of the things that are important to you? Or if you could remove the dross that clouds your relationships with friends, family, community and the environment you live in? The breath can be such a guide to this clarity of heart and mind. When you begin to see what is truly meaningful to you, you are no longer held captive by the dictates of those around you and can make choices that support your growing commitment to your welfare and the welfare of the world you live in. Your breathing can be an exquisite guide toward a way of being that is transformative not only for yourself but for all those that come into contact with you.

These next two breath meditations can be done as a part of a formal mindfulness practice, but they can also be used as little reminders throughout the day that may be only one breathcycle long. I often pause throughout my work day when I find my mind racing and my breathing accelerating and take one long breath in and out. When done with conscious awareness even these brief snatches can remind us that this moment is the only moment we have in which to live fully.

～ INQUIRY ～

The Breath of Birth and Death

(*A note*: I have always found this meditation profoundly relaxing and refreshing, but it is not unusual for people to find the idea of imagining their own death frightening and disturbing. If you find this exercise upsetting you are of course free to try another, but it may also be an interesting exercise to look more deeply at your fear of your own inevitable death. You might try imagining it to be a blissful relief and relaxation, as comforting as entering sleep after an exhausting day.)

Sit or lie down in a comfortable position. Take a moment to feel the newness of this moment. We take so much for granted in life. What a miracle it is to be alive and breathing! Now imagine that you have just been born and this is your very first breath. Imagine what it would have been like to take that first startling breath. Feel the sensation of the air entering your nostrils, cool and refreshing. As you do this, mentally say, "This is my first breath." Enjoy the feeling of the air filling and suffusing the chest. Imagine how each and every cell of your body is imbibing the life energy of the breath. Let the phrase reverberate inside you for a few minutes. Now as you breathe out imagine that this is your last breath. What will it be like to take your last precious breath? Try not to associate this with a gruesome accident but imagine this as a peaceful moment. As you do this, mentally say, "This is my last breath." Feel the breath leaving the body until the very last traces of the exhalation are gone from the lungs. Savor every moment of that breath. Now continue alternating the mental phrasing of "This is my first breath. This is my last breath," truly imagining what each would feel like. In truth each breath is our first breath, each breath is new and different and denotes a distinct moment in time. And none of us knows if today may be the last day that we draw breath. Can you breathe as if today were your last day on earth? Let the full meaning of this precious life suffuse you. Also feel the relief of letting the breath go and of resting in a state of repose. Continue with the internal chant as long as you like, taking a few minutes at the end to simply relax. As you continue with your day, stop every few hours and take a birthing breath and a dying breath. As you do this completely absorb everything that is happening to you.

What would your day look like if you knew this were your last day on earth? How would you spend your day? Keep in mind that you would not want to have any regrets or any ends left untied at the end of this day. Would it be possible to live each day with this same awareness?

～ INQUIRY ～

Entering the Stillness within the Breath

> *Are you looking for me?*
> *I am in the next seat.*
> *When you really look for me, you will see me*
> *instantly—*
> *you will find me in the tiniest house of time.*
> *Kabir says: Student, tell me, what is God?*
> *He is the breath inside the breath?*

—*KABIR*, VERSIONS BY ROBERT BLY

This meditation can be done sitting or lying down. First observe how your breath is coming and going, rising and falling. Like life, it is constantly changing. Where is the stillness, the ever-present, unchanging essence that lies at the root of all things? As you watch your breath in mindfulness practice, notice how the mind is captivated by thoughts, feelings and sensations. Notice how the mind can follow the endless fluctuations of the breath. Yet in between each breath there is a brief pause. It is most noticeable at the end of the exhalation. Allow your attention to be "captured" by this special pause between the rising and the falling of the breath. Feel yourself recline into that pause as if lying back into the arms of a someone you trusted with your life. Notice that in this pause there is no thought, no sensation—only a glistening stillness, pregnant with possibilities. As you enter the pause more completely, notice also that it becomes more spacious. As you feel the expanse of that pause let your whole being fill it. This is the root of the breath. The inhalation is born of this stillness and the exhalation returns to this stillness. Thoughts, feelings, and sensations, pleasant and unpleasant, arise and dissolve back into this unchanging stillness. Allow yourself to become this luminous stillness. Even as you witness the next movement of breath and the next movement of thought, witness it from the vantage point of that peaceful stillness. This stillness has always been present within you. As distractions arise, as noises and work projects assert their urgency upon your consciousness, there is no need to deflect or protect yourself from them—both stillness and thoughts can exist at the same time. Let yourself be nourished by the peace of this stillness and when you are ready open your eyes. Take a few moments to settle before you go on with your day. Carry this stillness with you throughout the day with each breath.

> Each breath is transforming me
> Into thine image.
>
> —J. KRISHNAMURTI

Merging with the Breath

I am conscious as this book comes to a close that all endings are in fact beginnings and that what we want in the end must be present in the beginning. The belief of some better or higher realm toward which we must stretch lies implicit in most of our religious and spiritual traditions. Thus for many of us, our self-reflective practice, whether it be a daily walk or a sitting meditation, can become yet another effort to reach this idealized goal. Just as our cultural myths act as an illusive oasis in the so-called desert of our present moment, we can fall into the same trap with a mindfulness practice. The danger is in thinking that through gradual improvement we will arrive one day as a truly perfect human being, and then, as we so often promise ourselves, we'll be happy. We may feel that we have a long road ahead of us. But we cannot progressively move toward knowing ourselves as we might know some object, because what we *are* and what we *wish to know* are not separate, but the same thing. We are this living, breathing, awakened Consciousness! The very nature of the breath arising from within us announces this message over and over again. And as yoga teacher and psychotherapist Richard Miller warns: "If we don't understand this simple fact, we may become ardent students of the breath, mastering long and complex breathing patterns and techniques, but miss the critical understanding toward which the breath is pointing. This attitude is tantamount to studying the finger and not seeing the moon toward which it points."[2]

This last inquiry brings us full circle back to the essential nature of the breath. As you have worked your way through each chapter you have learned to perceive and witness the life force of the breath as it moves through you. In witnessing your breath you may have experienced the breath as something separate from you. Ultimately, we are not separate from this life force, and thus this last inquiry involves a process of merging with the breath. This process of immersion, which is at once human and divine, is like merging with one's lover. When you first meet a beloved one you touch them, feel them, and take in everything about them with all your senses. You attempt to know them as separate from yourself. You may have searched far and wide in the hopes of finding this other person. But one day, you place your hands on the beloved and stay there for a long time. At first you do all the same things; feeling the texture of his skin, the perfume of her body, but as you stay and melt into this complete awareness of other, you notice that your perception of your hand and his body has merged, has become one unified body. In that moment you know yourself and you know the other as one. This is the same process by which we come to experience ourselves as wedded to the living, pulsing life force.

Let this last inquiry then be a beginning. As you feel compelled return to earlier inquiries in the book with this new awareness.

～ INQUIRY ～

Merging with the Breath

Sit or lie down in a comfortable position and become aware of your breathing. Feel your breath with all your senses; the sound of the breath as it enters and leaves the body, the sensation of coolness and warmth as it flows into and out of your nostrils, and the body visibly oscillating with every inspiration and expiration. As you palpate the breath with your awareness, allow whatever is arising on the current of the breath to come unimpeded and allow whatever is ebbing on the current of the breath to dissolve. Greet each new sensation, thought, feeling, or emotion with an open heart and mind. Welcome whatever the breath has to tell you.

Now feel yourself *as* the breath. Feel the breath as yourself arising and falling away, expanding and settling but always returning to the calm point of stillness. Let go of watching your breath and enter the breath with all your being and let yourself be entered by the breath. At first concentrate on the sensation of your own swelling and receding, ebbing and flowing, and the fluidity of this ever-changing movement of life force. Then gradually shift toward feeling yourself as the calm point of stillness from which the breath arises, from which you yourself arise in each moment. Allow yourself to become saturated with this stillness. Let yourself become this stillness that is your center. Even as you feel yourself arising and dissolving with each inhalation and exhalation, feel the stillness as ever present, ever enduring. Let yourself be penetrated by the completeness of this moment. Feel each breath as an announcement celebrating your own home-coming.

~ ~ ~

May each breath be like a footstep bringing you back to the home of yourself.

I have seen
A curious child, who dwelt upon a tract
of inland ground, applying to his ear
the convolutions of a smooth-lipped shell
To which, in silence hushed, his very soul
Listened intensely; and his countenance soon
Brightened with joy; for from within were heard
Murmurings, whereby the monitor expressed
Mysterious union with it's native sea.
Even such a shell the universe itself
Is to the ear of Faith; and there are times,
I doubt not, when to you it doth impart
Authentic tidings of invisible things;
Of ebb and flow, and ever-during power;
and central peace, subsisting at the heart
of endless agitation.

—FROM "*THE EXCURSION*,"
WILLIAM WORDSWORTH

Practice Guides

*N*ow that you have a repertoire of movements, inquiries, and breathing explorations you may want to incorporate them into some kind of daily "feel good" practice. This section is about taking the alphabet of what you've learned and making stories that work for your body and your specific needs. Generally, a breath work practice should consist of movements that open the body and stimulate your breathing followed by deep relaxation and a breathing inquiry of your choice. You can choose from the many movements you learned in chapter 5 as well as the breathing inquiries in chapter 6 to design a program that meets your needs. Don't feel compelled to stick to a formal practice structure; use the exercises creatively.

If you don't feel confident putting together your own program, you can try the suggested "Feel Good" programs below. They take about 30 minutes each. Once you've learned Programs A, B, and C you can alternate them throughout the week, or you can focus on one program for weeks or even months at a time. If you haven't the time to do an entire program in one session, consider dividing the program into a morning and evening session. Or you may want to focus on the practice sessions designed for retraining specific breath holding patterns. Although having a formal practice can be important for establishing and sustaining your sense of well-being and vitality, don't ignore the "rest" of the day, which can offer an opportunity to integrate what you have learned about breathing. In this way, all of life can become a practice of growing awareness.

GENERAL "FEEL GOOD" PROGRAMS

PROGRAM A (WEEKS 1–2)

1. Tapping and Percussion with the Lion Pose page 115, Fig. 17 & 18
2. Breath Stretches page 117, Fig. 19A, B & C
3. Roll Downs page 118, Fig. 20A & B
4. Shoulder Clock page 130, Fig. 26
5. Diaphragm Release A page 134, Fig. 29A
6. Pelvic and Hip Openers page 124, Fig. 23A, B, C & D
7. Effortless Rest position: Practice page 18, Fig. 3
8. Choose one breath exercise from the following and focus on it for the first few weeks or alternate the selections:
   - Diaphragmatic Breathing A (7 minutes) page 150, Fig. 33A
   - Sandbag Breathing (10 minutes) page 151, Fig. 33B
   - Sounding the Exhalation (5–10 minutes) page 155

PROGRAM B (WEEKS 3–4)

1. Roll Downs page 118, Fig. 20A & B
2. Shoulder Clock page 130, Fig. 26
3. Shoulder and Upper Back Release page 131, Fig. 27
4. The Cat: Variation A & B page 120, Fig. 21A & B
5. Diaphragm Release B page 135, Fig. 29B
6. Pelvic and Hip Openers page 124, Fig. 23B, C, D, & E
7. The Waterfall with Guiding Relaxation page 137, Fig. 30B
   - Following the Lure of the Breath page 143
8. Revolved Belly Pose page 127, Fig. 24
9. Breathing Easy position page 141, Fig. 32

Choose one of the following:
   - Straw Breathing (5–10 minutes) page 152, Fig. 34
   - The Three-Part Breath (10 minutes) page 156

PROGRAM C (WEEKS 5–6)

1. Tapping and Percussion with the Lion Pose page 115, Fig. 17 & 18
2. Breath Stretches page 117, Fig. 19A, B & C
3. The Cat: Variation A & B page 120, Fig. 21A & B
4. Gateway Pose page 133, Fig. 28
5. Pelvic and Hip Openers page 124, Fig. 23A
5. Pelvic and Hip Openers page 124, Fig. 23B, C, D, & E
6. Supported Bound Angle page 128, Fig. 25
7. Effortless Rest position with your choice of guided relaxation.

You can do your breathing inquiries reclining or change to a sitting position. Choose one from the following:
- Alternate Nostril Breathing with counting (10 minutes) page 161, Fig. 35
- Merging with the Breath page 196

GUIDES FOR DEALING WITH SPECIFIC BREATH HOLDING PATTERNS

In chapter 4 you may have identified a specific breath holding pattern on which you would like to focus. Each program should take about 20–40 minutes if done in succession. Because breath holding patterns involve the entire body it's important also to have a more global approach so take the time to explore *all* the movements in chapter 5 and make your own choices about which ones work best for you.

REVERSE BREATHING

Do These Inquiries First:

∼ Inquiry: Checking In with Your Breath page 15
∼ Inquiry: The Marriage of Breath and Movement page 16, Fig. 1 & 2

Practice Sequence:

1. Pelvic and Hip Openers page 124, Fig. 23A, B, C, D, E
2. Supported Bound Angle page 128, Fig. 25
3. Revolved Belly Pose page 127, Fig. 24
4. Breathing Easy Pose: Choose one of the guided relaxations.

CHEST BREATHING

Practice Sequence:

1. Shoulder Clock page 130, Fig. 26
2. Shoulder and Upper Back Release page 131, Fig. 27
3. Diaphragm Release Variation A and B page 134, Fig. 29 A & B
4. Pelvic and Hip Openers page 124, Fig. 23A, B, C, D, E
5. Supported Bound Angle page 128, Fig. 25
6. Revolved Belly Pose page 127, Fig. 24
7. The Waterfall page 137, Fig. 30B
8. Effortless Rest position page 18, Fig. 3
9. Choose one of the following breath inquiries:
   - Straw Breathing (5–10 minutes) page 152, Fig. 34
   - Lengthening the Exhalation (5–10 minutes) page 102
   - The Three-Part Breath (5–10 minutes) page 156

COLLAPSED BREATHING

Practice Sequence:

1. Tapping and Percussion page 115, Fig. 17
2. Lion Pose page 115, Fig. 18
3. Roll Downs page 118, Fig. 20A & B
4. Breath Stretches page 117, Fig. 19A to C
5. Shoulder Clock page 130, Fig. 26
6. Shoulder and Upper Back Release page 131, Fig. 27
7. Diaphragm Release A & B page 134, Fig. 29A & B
8. The Waterfall page 137, Fig. 30B

9. Breathing Easy position page 141, Fig. 32
10. Choose one of the breathing inquiries:
    - Kapalabhati Cleansing Breath (10 rounds) page 158
    - Sandbag Breathing (5–10 minutes) page 151, Fig. 35

HYPERVENTILATION

Practice Sequence:

1. Roll Downs page 118, Fig. 20A & B
2. Shoulder Clock page 130, Fig. 26
3. Shoulder and Upper Back Release page 131, Fig. 27
4. Diaphragm Release A & B page 134, Fig. 29A & B
5. Pelvic and Hip Openers page 124, Fig. 23A, B, C, D, & E
6. Revolved Belly Pose page 127, Fig. 24
7. Supported Bound Angle page 128, Fig. 25
8. Supported Child's Pose page 140, Fig. 31
9. The Waterfall page 137, Fig. 30B
10. Effortless Rest position page 18, Fig. 3
11. Choose one of the following breath inquiries:
    - Lengthening the Exhalation page 102
    - The Three-Part Breath page 156
    - Straw Breathing page 152, Fig. 34

THROAT HOLDING

Practice Sequence:

1. Tapping and Percussion page 115, Fig. 17
2. Lion's Pose page 115, Fig. 18
3. Shoulder Clock page 130, Fig. 26
4. Diaphragm Release B page 135, Fig. 29A & B
5. The Waterfall page 137, Fig. 30B
6. Breathing Easy position while doing: page 141, Fig. 32
    - Sounding the Exhalation page 155

BREATH GRABBING

Breath Grabbing usually goes hand in hand with Chest Breathing and Hyperventilation. Refer to these sections for recommendations.

FROZEN BREATHING

First Read:

BodyBreath Synchrony page 110, Illustrations 28 and 29

Practice Sequence:

1. Roll Downs page 118, Fig. 20A & B
2. Shoulder Clock page 130, Fig. 26
3. Shoulder and Upper Back Release page 131, Fig. 27
4. The Cat (especially the variation with a partner) page 120, Fig. 21 & 22
5. Gateway Pose page 133, Fig. 28
6. Diaphragm Release A & B page 134, Fig. 29A & B
7. Pelvic and Hip Openers page 124, Fig. 23A, B, C, D, & E
8. Revolved Belly Pose page 127, Fig. 24
9. The Waterfall page 137, Fig. 30B
10. Breathing Easy position
11. One of the following relaxations or breath inquiries:
    - Strengthening Diaphragmatic Breathing A page 149, Fig. 33A
    - Sandbag Breathing page 151, Fig. 33B

GUIDES FOR HEALTH CONDITIONS AND SPECIFIC INTERESTS

The health conditions I have presented are complex subjects that would require an entire book (or collection of books) to cover sufficiently. I encourage you to do your own research, especially with regard to dietary, medical, and alternative health therapies that may be appropriate for your particular problem. It is rare for any condition to respond to only one approach for it cannot usually be attributed to one, single thing. Breathing, as well as diet, lifestyle, exercise, and numerous other factors need to be taken into consideration when contemplating treatment for a health condition. Because of this, the sequence guide is limited to ways in which breathing may help these conditions, and is not intended to imply that breath work should be your only line of action.

Others of you may feel motivated to use breath work to hone your concentration, heighten your sexual pleasure, or improve your athletic performance. These, as well as other practical applications for breath work are addressed in this section.

In all the practice guides, I have suggested specific inquiries and sections of the book that you may want to review for your particular area of interest. Take the time to reread these sections and familiarize yourself with the inquiries before doing the practice session. The exercises and inquiries are presented in a sequence that will make sense to your body rather than in the order in which they appear in the book.

Caution: The suggestions below are not meant as a replacement for necessary medical treatment and should be discontinued immediately if they cause your condition to worsen.

Allergies (see Headaches and/or Sinusitis)

Arthritis

Most arthritic conditions respond well to gentle exercise, especially when the exercise is non–weight bearing. Those that suffer from this disease find that the more they move, the more their condition improves. Swimming is a particularly good exercise for those with arthritis because it is non–weight bearing and strengthens the entire respiratory and circulatory system. Even those who are confined to bed or wheelchairs, however, can take advantage of the internal massage that occurs during deep breathing. Slow and deep breathing has also been shown to decrease pain levels and increase coping skills.

Do These Inquiries First

∼ Inquiry: The Marriage of Breath and Movement (Keep the movements small and relaxed) page 16, Fig. 1 & 2
∼ Inquiry: Organ Breathing page 100

Practice Sequence (20–30 minutes)

1. Breath Stretches page 117, Fig. 19A, B & C
2. Shoulder Clock (move far enough away from the wall to prevent shoulder compression) page 130, Fig. 26
3. Shoulder and Upper Back Release page 131, Fig. 27
4. The Cat (if you cannot bear weight on your wrists, try resting on your forearms) page 120, Fig. 21A & B
5. Pelvic and Hip Openers page 124, Fig. 23A to D
6. The Waterfall page 137, Fig. 30B

Choose one from the following:
- Sandbag Breathing page 151, Fig. 33B
- The Three-Part Breath page 15

Asthma

Asthma is a reversible lung disease that is characterized by hyperirritability of the bronchial airways. An attack, triggered by any number of environmental or emotional stressors, is characterized by inflammation, constriction, and spasm of the airways, and increased secretion of mucus by the bronchi. These physiological changes cause the wheezing, coughing, and shortness of breath so familiar to asthma sufferers.

Some of the common features of a typical asthmatic's breathing pattern are:

- Premature curtailing of the exhalation, with use of the secondary respiratory muscles to initiate inhalation. As a result these accessory muscles in the upper chest, back, and neck become overdeveloped.

- Loss of the normal pause at the end of the exhalation. Medical researchers have indicated that learning to allow the inhalation to spontaneously grow out of this pause is the key to restoring normal diaphragmatic breathing.[1]

- Poor posture, characterized by a rounding of the upper back (kyphosis) which may be accompanied by a flattening of the lumbar curve (hypolordosis) and shortening of the abdominal muscles. These changes make normal diaphragmatic breathing difficult.

- A vicious cycle created by these abnormal breathing habits contributing to both anxiety and the continuation of asthmatic symptoms.[2]

Yoga and yogic breathing practices have been shown to relieve many of these symptoms. One study on treating asthma patients with yogic practices, conducted by researchers John Goyeche, Dr. Ago, and Dr. Ikemi, suggests that any effective treatment should address suppressed emotions—such as anxiety and self-image—as well as the physical dimension. To achieve this they encourage correction of poor posture, and helping the person to relax the irrelevant respiratory muscles, while restoring full diaphragmatic breathing. They also recommended finding ways for getting rid of excess mucus.[3] The good news is that a well-rounded breath work practice will do all these things.

Numerous other scientifically controlled experiments showed that regular deep breathing exercises combined with yoga postures and meditation could diminish the frequency of asthma attacks, the need for medication (and in some cases eliminate the need for medical treatment altogether), increase lung capacity, slow the breathing rate, and calm the central nervous system.[4]

Other practices that may be helpful are swimming (if you are not too debilitated) and regular walking. Graduate your walking from a normal to brisk pace always ending with walking the last few blocks at very slow pace. Graduate from walking on flat ground to more difficult terrain including hills and stairs. Increase the length of your walks and the speed of your walking only if this does not promote asthmatic conditions. Never get so "puffed" that you can't hold a comfortable conversation.

Read

- Chest or Paradoxical Breathing page 77

Do These Inquiries First

- ～ Inquiry: Movements of the Breath page 24
- ～ Inquiry: Where Do I Breathe? page 36
- ～ Inquiry: The Dance of the Diaphragms page 60

Practice Sequence (40–60 minutes)

1. Tapping and Percussion★ with the Lion page 115, Fig. 17 & 18
2. Shoulder Clock page 130, Fig. 26
3. The Cat: Variation A page 12, Fig. 21A & B
4. Shoulder and Upper Back Release page 131, Fig. 27
5. Gateway Pose page 133, Fig. 28
6. Diaphragm Release A & B★★ (1–3 minutes each) page 134, Fig. 29A & B
7. Waterfall★★★ (5–10 minutes) page 137, Fig. 30B
8. Assume the Breathing Easy position for all Relaxation and Breath Exercises.

Choose one from the following list:
- Following the Lure of the Breath page 143
- Strengthening Diaphragmatic Breathing; pick the one you enjoy the most (5–10 minutes) page 149
- Straw Breathing (5–10 minutes) page 152, Fig. 34

Back Pain (refer to **Pain Relief**)

Childbirth

Many of my students who have taken yoga classes with me throughout their second pregnancies have reported that their new-found awareness of the pelvic diaphragm and of their breathing in general, made for a shorter and easier labor.

★ Tapping and percussion is particularly important to loosen mucus so it can be expelled. This can be made doubly effective if you have a friend tap your lower lung area, both in the front and back, while you have your *head lower than your chest*. You can do this by lying on your side with a pillow elevating your lower lung, or by resting in the Waterfall position. In the latter position it's easy to tap the lungs by yourself.

★★ These back bending movements may elicit the same sensation of constriction in the chest that asthmatics associate with an impending attack. If you find this scary or uncomfortable, try lowering the height of the prop. See if you can relax into the movement by taking long breaths out through your mouth with pursed lips. Gradually increase the diameter of the prop as you feel more confident in opening the chest.

★★★ The Waterfall is an extraordinary posture for asthmatics. If you have time for no other practice do this one! Inversion of the lungs causes the diaphragm to ascend, with gravity assisting full exhalation. The position of the abdominal organs allows the diaphragm to spontaneously open and the inversion helps to drain the lungs of fluid. This pose has a deep calming effect on the nervous system, which may help to reset some of the autonomic responses that cause the hyperirritability of the bronchioles in the first place.

These women also commented on how they felt more in tune with the process because they knew how to let their breathing spontaneously change in response to pain and exhaustion. I have since come to the conclusion a greater understanding of their breathing and the movements that occur in the pelvis and lower abdomen can be invaluable to a woman in childbirth.

There are differing opinions about the efficacy of using specific breathing patterns during birthing. I tend to agree with Carl Jones, author of *Alternative Birth,* who feels that concentrating on any one set pattern of breathing can "interfere with a spontaneous response to labor and can actually impede labor's progress."[5] He also found that bedside fathers often became so focused on coaching a set breathing pattern that they tended to neglect more effective means of labor support, such as massaging the laboring woman or providing verbal encouragement. It seems clear that since most of us breathe poorly and we tend to meet difficulty with tension rather than relaxation, a heightened *awareness* of breathing gives a woman the ability to respond both spontaneously and intelligently to the challenge of her child's birth.

If you feel that learning a breathing technique would give you confidence, many current authorities on birth training now recommend the Bradley Method, a system that teaches slow breathing rather than the shallow, panting breathing characteristic of the Lamaze method. Rapid chest breathing can lead to hyperventilation, a condition that will make you feel light-headed and even numb in your hands and fingers. This isn't good for you or for your baby. If during particularly heavy contractions you have breathed so rapidly that you begin to feel the symptoms of hyperventilation, take a long and slow breath *out* and immediately your next breath will be fuller. This slow diaphragmatic breathing can provide a focal point for your concentration when the going gets rough.

During the second stage of labor women are often encouraged to push strenuously during contractions—which many women accomplish by holding their breath. Breath holding during the second stage has been associated with a drop in fetal heart rates and a concomitant reduction in the fetal oxygen supply.[6] Despite our cultural predilection to treat birth as a competitive athletic event (with a speedy birth considered a successful one), studies show that when woman are allowed to follow their own inclinations they are able to deliver as quickly as mothers that were actively encouraged to push.[7] They also reduced their chances of tearing and requiring an episiotomy by up to 40 percent. Rahima Baldwin, author of *Special Delivery,* advises pushing only when there is an "irresistible urge" to do so and suggests that when you feel the need, you help your body push effectively by *expanding out* through your lower belly and perineum. She adds, "Most of us, when we think of pushing as in having a bowel movement, think of pushing *in* on the belly as we hold our breath. This is just the opposite of what you need to do in second stage to birth your baby. Your baby's head requires that everything down below is open and stretches as the head bulges forward on your perineal tissue.[8] Remember, when you breathe in fully and allow your belly to expand the diaphragm presses downward, which can only help the birthing process.

In the Physiologic Approach to the second stage of labor (a modern approach that is actually a return to older midwife wisdom), the mother is "encouraged to breathe spontaneously while keeping her mouth open, relaxing her jaw and throat, and making as much noise as she likes." She is also cautioned "to avoid cutting off the flow of breath, as an open glottis (throat) is associated with opening in the pelvic and vaginal areas."[9]

All of these approaches reflect the basic belief that it can be a trap to go into labor with a set idea about how it should progress and a prescribed way of breathing throughout. While following a technique may give you confidence, it can also prevent you from making choices in response to what is actually happening (rather than what you imagined *should* happen). These choices also include letting your breathing change in response to your body's cues.

Regardless of the particular approach you choose for your labor, it will be crucial to remain attentive to what is happening rather than being overwhelmed with fear or panic. Your breathing can act as a palpable lifeline to keep you tethered to the present moment. If you have a heightened awareness of your body and the effects that different body positions and breathing techniques have on you personally, you will be better able to respond to what is happening and to ask for what you need, whether that be a change of position or more support from your partner. As one of my students said, "During my first labor I didn't even know where my perineum was or how to breathe in such a way as to open rather than close there. During my second labor, I knew not only where to open but how to do it, and I felt I could trust my body because it was a body I *knew* rather than a stranger to me."

Read

The Pelvic Diaphragm see page 54, Illustration 15

Do These Inquiries First

∼ Inquiry: Movements of the Breath (focus on the pelvis, sacral, and lower back movements) page 24, Illustrations 1 & 2

Preliminary Caution:

After the third month of pregnancy you should do all supine breathing exercises in the Breathing Easy position (see page 137, Fig. 32) with sufficient propping to raise your heart above the level of your abdomen. Do your relaxation in the alternative side-lying position (see page 29, Fig. 6). Lying on your back can interfere with the blood supply to the fetus (and to yourself), as the weight of the baby presses against the inferior vena cava (the blood vessel that returns blood from the lower body to the heart). Elevating the torso at an angle will prevent this and also open the area around the diaphragm, reducing common symptoms such as heartburn and indigestion.

Important Note: In many inquiries I have elaborated on the importance of relaxing the pelvic floor during inhalation. Learning to relax the pelvic floor can help a woman immeasurably during the second and final stages of labor when this area must expand radically to accommodate the baby's head. However, at no time is there greater pressure on the pelvic floor, or greater risk of these important muscles being damaged, than during pregnancy. Pelvic exercises that tone and strengthen these muscles can help maintain the pelvic floor during pregnancy and can reestablish integrity in the postpartum pelvic floor. Speedy deliveries, long second stage labor (where the baby's head is pressing against the perineum), and poorly repaired episiotomies can all cause extensive damage to the pelvic floor muscles, affecting a woman's continence. For this reason, you would be advised to follow the recommendations of your midwife or consulting gynecologist or obstetrician on how to do effective pelvic floor exercises. Biofeedback studies have shown that many woman who believe they are doing pelvic floor exercises are using other muscles instead, so you may want to seek professional advice to check if you are doing the exercises correctly.

Practice Sequence: Prenatal (30 minutes)

1. Breath Stretches page 117, Fig. 19A, B & C
2. Shoulder Clock page 130, Fig. 26

3. Shoulder and Upper Back Release page 131, Fig. 27
4. The Cat: Variation A page 120, Fig. 21A & B
5. Pelvic and Hip Openers (first trimester only) page 124, Fig. 23 A & B only
   After the first trimester try Squatting instead page 33
6. Supported Bound Angle: raise the body up to 45 degrees or until comfortable (5–10 minutes) page 128, Fig. 25
7. Assume the Breathing Easy position (with extra propping so the body is at a 30–40 degree angle) for the following breathing inquiries. Or you can sit. Choose one of the following to end your session:
   - Strengthening Diaphragmatic Breathing: Variation A page 149, Fig. 33A
   - Lengthening the Exhalation page 102
   - Sounding the Exhalation page 155

Concentration: Building Mind Stamina

Breathing is the bridge to the mind. Of all the techniques below I find the alternate nostril breathing one of the quickest and most dramatic techniques for focusing the mind. Experiment with each technique to see how it works for you in different situations so you'll have options to pick from your hat of breath tricks.

Practice Sequence (10–15 minutes)

1. Clear the nose with a nasal wash each morning page 64
2. Following the Lure of the Breath (10 minutes) page 143
3. Choose one of the following:

   - Straw Breathing (5–15 minutes) page 152, Fig. 34
   - Alternate Nostril Breathing: Either variation (5–15 minutes) page 161, Fig. 35

Constipation

Constipation is frequently the result of ignoring the call of nature. When the body sends us the message that we need to go to the bathroom, the first signal is the strongest. If we ignore this first signal, the contraction of the colon will not be as strong later. While low dietary fiber, inadequate water intake, and irregular exercise can contribute to constipation, chronic tightening of the abdomen prevents the entire digestive track from receiving the deep stimulating massage of the breath. Entire aisles in our nation's drugstores are devoted to laxative formulas, which may be more a testimony to "tight ass" breathing than to any other cause. When you do heed the call of nature, instead of bearing down, which can create hemorrhoids, focus on deep relaxed belly breathing. Often, only a few minutes of patient breathing will stimulate the bowel.

Read

- Chest or Paradoxical Breathing page 77, Illustrations 21 and 22
- Two Myths About Your Belly page 39

Do These Inquiries First

～ Inquiry: Organ Breathing (focus on breathing into your lower abdomen) page 100, Illustration 12

Practice Sequence:

1. Pelvic and Hip Openers page 124, Fig. 23A to D
2. Revolved Belly Pose (two repetitions each side) page 127, Fig. 24
3. The Waterfall page 137, Fig. 30B
4. Choose one of the following breathing exercises:
   - Sandbag Breathing (5–10 minutes) page 151, Fig. 33B
   - The Three-Part Breath page 152
5. Walk for at least 30 minutes three times a week

(Note: If you lack tone in the abdomen, for one week try doing a morning and afternoon practice of Kapalabhati for 3–4 rounds. This will help stimulate bowel contractions and tone of the entire abdomen page 158)

Depression

Depression creates a feeling of inertia, as if gravity were somehow strongest over the place that we inhabit. Because of the power of this inertia, movement—*any movement*—can be helpful in breaking free. I strongly recommend a brisk daily walk, preferably vigorous, of at least 30 minutes, where you *must* breathe more deeply. Bicycling, swimming, or doing a yoga practice can also be very helpful. Move strongly enough so that your breathing has to deepen but don't ever get so puffed that you can't keep up a conversation. The movements in this practice sequence focus on enlivening and quickening the breathing and body.

Moving or engaging in an activity as a way to break out of the inertia of depression should not be mistaken for running away from the cause of your depression. If this is your tendency it may be better for you to do a deeply soothing and relaxing practice where you can get in touch with the feelings underneath the depression. Try the "Fatigue/Recuperation from Illness" sequence instead. If your depression is seriously debilitating, consider seeking the help of a qualified professional.

Practice Sequence (30–40 minutes)

1. Begin with nasal wash to clear your head page 64
2. Tapping and percussion (preferably in fresh air) page 115, Fig. 18 & 19
3. Kapalabhati (3–5 minutes) page 158
4. Breath Stretches page 117, Fig. 19A, B & C
5. Roll Downs page 118, Fig. 20A & B
6. Shoulder Clock page 131, Fig. 26
7. Shoulder and Upper Back Release page 131, Fig. 26
8. Diaphragm Release B page 135, Fig. 29B
9. The Waterfall page 137, Fig. 30B
10. Choose one of the following to end your practice:
    • Sandbag Breathing (5 minutes) page 151, Fig. 33B
    • Sounding the Exhalation (5 minutes) page 155
    • Alternate Nostril Breathing with counting (5 minutes) page 161, Fig. 36

Eating Disorders (anorexia nervosa, chronic dieting, bulimia, obesity)

Although you may not categorize yourself as someone who suffers from an eating disorder, the sheer weight of statistics on obesity and dieting speak of a nation obsessed with the issue of food and body image. Having personally had anorexia during my late adolescence and early twenties, I feel particularly sensitive to the way eating disorders shape breathing. Contracting throughout the abdomen or alternately collapsing the abdomen seem to be common breath holding strategies for people with eating disorders. The desire to look thin eclipses the need to breathe. This conflict also plays itself out during meal times when you may tighten your stomach and diaphragm area, making the motions of ingesting food while "refusing" it at the same time with the body. This refusal is taken a step further by a bulimic who will vomit so frequently that her teeth may be permanently eroded from acid damage. The subconscious refusal to take nourishment may continue long after eating is over (often experienced as regret or shame for having eaten at all), so that over time the breath is constricted all the time. Being aware of these holding patterns, especially as they crop up before, during, and after eating, can be particularly powerful in facing and resolving the conflict that arises around nourishment of the self.

On yoga retreats participants often join me in a "breath lunch." Try this during any meal by yourself (preferably where you can eat in silence). Observe how you breathe as you eat and make sure you are not holding your abdomen and stomach area tight during the meal. You may find, as my retreat guests do, that you eat less, enjoy your food more, digest your food better, and can respond to the message from your stomach, "I am *almost* full," by putting your fork down.

Read

• Two Myths About Your Belly page 39

Do These Inquiries First

∼ Inquiry: Chest or Paradoxical Breathing page 77,
   Illustrations 21 & 22
∼ Inquiry: Contracting Your Diaphragm page 73

Practice Sequence (40 minutes)

1. Shoulder and Upper Back Release page 131, Fig. 27
2. Pelvic and Hip Openers page 124, Fig. 23A, B, C, D, E & F
3. Revolved Belly Pose page 127, Fig. 24
4. Diaphragm Release Variation A and B page 134, Fig. 29 A & B
5. The Waterfall page 137, Fig. 30B
6. Relaxation: Supported Child's Pose page 140, Fig. 31
7. Do one of the following to end your practice session:
    • Organ Breathing (focus on your belly for 10 minutes) page 100, Illustration 12
    • Three-Part Breath (5–10 minute) page 156

- Sounding the Exhalation (5–10 minutes) page 155
- Alternate Nostril Breathing (use this when you feel the urge to binge or when you feel tension before a meal) page 161, Fig. 35

Enhancing Sexual Pleasure

This section focuses on opening and releasing tension in the pelvic area. Enhancing sexual pleasure, however, involves living and inhabiting all of the body, not only the few square inches around the genitals. If you are a couple wanting to explore more extensively, please refer to chapter 7: The Shared Breath.

Some of you may have turned to this section because you are dealing with more serious sexual issues. Breath work can be very powerful for helping release long suppressed feelings and for increasing the vitality in previously numb or unresponsive areas of the body. This can be an exciting process but it can also be painful and difficult. I recommend to my own clients that they work in tandem with a professional therapist if they have serious sexual issues.

Read

The Pelvic Diaphragm page 54, Illustration 15

Do These Inquiries First

～ Inquiry: The Movements of the Breath (focus on the pelvic floor, sacrum, and lumbar spine areas, especially in squatting) page 24, Illustrations 6 & 7.
～ Inquiry: The Dance of the Diaphragms page 60, Illustration 13 & 14

Practice Sequence (30–40 minutes)

1. Pelvic and Hip Openers page 124, Fig. 23A, B, C & D
2. Revolved Belly Pose page 127, Fig. 24
3. Supported Bound Angle page 128, Fig. 25
4. Diaphragm Release A & B page 134, Fig. 29A & B
5. Supported Child's Pose page 140, Fig. 31
6. Choose one of the following:
   - Kapalabhati (5–10 minutes to increase sensation in the lower body) page 158
   - Organ Breathing (focus on breathing into abdominal area) page 100, Illustration 12

- Strengthening Diaphragmatic Breathing A page 149, Fig. 33A
- The Three-Part Breath (to gradually relax body armoring) page 156

Fatigue/Recuperation from Illness

There is a distinct difference between mental lethargy and true physical fatigue. To determine whether you are physically tired try practicing a few movements (or whatever exercise you like) and if you feel your fatigue worsen switch to something more passive and regenerative. If your energy starts to lift you've probably been feeling mental lassitude. Sometimes what we most need at the end of the work day (especially if our work is intellectual and sedentary) is to get moving. If you think this is the case for you, refer to the practice sequence for Depression, which focuses on enlivening the breathing and body.

If you have chronic fatigue syndrome, or a medical problem such as an auto immune disease in which fatigue is a major symptom, be careful not to tire yourself in your practice, especially when doing the breathing exercises. When recovering from an illness, even if it's just a cold, it can be very discouraging to remember what you could do before you got sick, or how much stamina you used to have. There's a tendency to use this past measure as a reference point and to do too much too soon, often resulting in a relapse. Focus instead on improving the quality of how you feel, rather than on how many repetitions you do or how long you stay in the different movements.

Practice Sequence (30–40 minutes)

1. Pelvic and Hip Openers page 124, Fig. 23A, B, C & D
2. Revolved Belly Pose page 127, Fig. 24
3. Supported Bound Angle page 128, Fig. 25
4. Diaphragm Release A & B page 134, Fig. 29A & B
5. The Waterfall (10 minutes) page 137, Fig. 30B
6. Breathing Easy position page 141, Fig. 32
7. Choose one of the following breathing inquiries:
   - Strengthening Diaphragmatic Breathing A & B page 149, 33 A & B
   - Alternate Nostril Breathing (5–10 minutes) page 161, Fig. 35

Headaches

Headaches have many causes, from allergies and eye strain to compression in the neck and serious organic problems such as spinal infections. Headaches are also a specific symptom of hyperventilation, and people commonly notice the onset of a headache when they are feeling particularly stressed. If you have chronic headaches, you owe it to yourself to get a full physical checkup from your health practitioner. He or she may be able to help you identify a causative factor that you can rectify.

A recent University of Pittsburgh Medical Center study of women who had relied on prescription medication to control chronic tension or migraine headaches until they became pregnant, showed that 80 percent of them experienced fewer and less intense headaches after only four sessions of biofeedback training focusing on deep breathing. They were also able to maintain the improvement at home without biofeedback equipment. The following practice session focuses on breathing into the abdominal area and relaxing the head, neck, and shoulder area. It is generally not a good idea to invert the body if you *already* have a headache.

Read

- Chest or Paradoxical Breathing page 77, Illustrations 21 and 22
- Hyperventilation page 83

Do These Inquiries First

- ～ Inquiry: Back Breathing page 98, Fig. 16
- ～ Inquiry: Soft Eyes/Open Diaphragm page 103

Practice Sequence (30 minutes)

1. Pelvic and Hip Openers page 124, Fig. 23A, B, C & D
2. Revolved Belly Pose page 127, Fig. 24
3. Supported Bound Angle page 128, Fig. 25
4. Shoulder and Upper Back Release on chair page 131, Fig. 27
5. Breathing Easy position (cover the eyes and forehead with an ace bandage wound *lightly* around the head. This will block out light, deeply relax all the muscles in the face and eyes, and elicit deep relaxed breathing)

6. Choose one of the following:
   - Lengthening the Exhalation page 102
   - The Three-Part Breath page 156

(Imagine the brain shrinking away from the walls of the skull on each successive exhalation)

Improving Athletic Performance (running, cycling, and swimming)

Although athletes and their trainers gave little attention to breathing in the past, breathing techniques are now becoming an integral part of sports training. Doctor and triathlete John Hellemans (ranked first in the world in his age group) recommends that the best breathing for top athletic performance is deep diaphragmatic breathing. Studies with asthmatics have shown that an increase in the excursion of the diaphragm increases lung capacity. Dr. Hellemans also notes the importance of getting into a rhythmic flow with your breathing and synchronizing your breathing with your movement. You can do that by taking a breath when you plant your foot during a stride, when pedaling on a cycle, or when you stroke the water in the pool. Find a rhythm and speed of movement that allows you to work *within the confines of your breath capacity,* so that you are not building up an oxygen deficit.

Keep in mind, too, that one of the main differences between an average and extraordinary athlete may be sheer lung capacity. While lung capacity can be improved, much of our physiology may be inherited. Sabino Padilla, the doctor and physiologist for Miguel Indurain, five-time winner of the Tour de France, explains that the Spaniard's lung capacity is a huge factor in his success. While the average cyclist or marathon runner can take in only six liters of air, Indurain can take in eight.[10]

Most of us, however, aren't competing at such levels of performance. But whether it is a daily run, weekend hiking, or a thrice weekly swim, establishing a diaphragmatic breath and maintaining low breathing will help you enhance your performance. In one case study, a strong swimmer who could do all strokes except freestyle was taught diaphragmatic breathing. Before the training she experienced shortness of breath and feelings of panic after only 50 meters (one length) of freestyle. After four weeks of practicing diaphragmatic breathing both in and out of the water, the same woman was able to swim 40 lengths without any symptoms of breathlessness. Because the woman had been a strong swimmer to begin with, her improvement is most likely attributed to the shift in her breathing pattern rather than to a general improvement in fitness levels.[11]

If you want to maximize your athletic workouts, consider interval training. This involves alternating maximum-paced work with slower paced work. Those that used interval training increased their oxygen uptake by 11 to 18 percent over a twelve-week period while those that slogged along at the same pace showed little improvement or remained the same.

Regardless of your physical activity, you always want to assume a body posture that puts the diaphragm in an optimal position to breathe. If you tire easily, examine your posture carefully. This means not hunching over your handlebars on the bike, but opening the space between the tip of your breastbone and your belly. For runners, it means not tilting forward with the shoulders and over-tightening the abdominal muscles. The following practice is designed for pre-athletic activity. The focus is on stretching the diaphragm and entraining diaphragmatic breathing so it can become an automatic habit when you exercise.

Read

The Diaphragm page 52, Illustration 11
Breathing and the Heart page 59
The Lower Lungs page 65

Do These Inquiries First

～ Inquiry: Contracting Your Diaphragm page 73
～ Inquiry: The Dance of the Diaphragms page 60,
   Illustrations 13 & 14
～ Inquiry: Soft Eyes/Open Diaphragm page 103
(This technique is extremely effective for interactive group sports in which you want to be very aware of your surroundings and the other people around you.)

Practice Sequence (30 minutes)

1. Tapping and Percussion with the Lion Pose page 115, Fig. 17 & 18
2. Kapalabhati (3 rounds) page 158
3. Breath Stretches page 118, Fig. 19A, B, and C
4. Shoulder Clock page 131, Fig. 26

5. Gateway Pose page 133, Fig. 28
6. Diaphragm Release A & B page 134, Fig. 29A & B
7. Breathing Easy position page 141, Fig. 32
8. Choose one of the following to finish:
   - Sandbag Breathing (5–10 minutes) page 151, Fig. 33B
   - Alternate Nostril Breathing (for increasing concentration and reducing nervousness before an event, especially one requiring skillful coordination such as gymnastics) page 161, Fig. 35

Insomnia

When insomnia is caused by an overactive or worried mind, you'll find that your breathing speeds up or becomes erratic. Get into the habit of making the last hour before sleep a quiet, reflective time. Don't watch action-packed TV, see violent films, or engage in challenging intellectual problem-solving right before bed. This will only insure that your sleep (if you even get to sleep) will be restless. The following practice is designed to be done before bed. Do it in your nightclothes and close to your bed, so that you can easily slide into bed for the final relaxation.

Practice Sequence (15 minutes)

1. Diaphragm Release: A page 134, Fig. 29A
2. The Waterfall (Cover the eyes and forehead with an ace bandage wound *lightly* around the head and keep it on while you fall asleep. You could also cover your eyes with an eye bag.) page 137, Fig. 30B
3. Now climb into bed and lie on your back with a pillow under your knees. Practice the breath work until you begin to feel drowsy, then release any control of your breath and let yourself drift off to sleep. Choose one from the following:

   - Experiencing the Essential Breath page 9
   - Lengthening the Exhalation page 102
   - The Three-Part Breath (this is particularly powerful when you also visualize layers of tension dropping away with each successive exhalation page 156

Menopausal Hot Flashes

Recent studies have shown that women who practice deep, slow diaphragmatic breathing can reduce the frequency of hot flashes. This practice session focuses on increasing the circulation around the sex organs and cooling the body. If you are very tired, use the Fatigue practice sequence, page 217.

Practice Sequence (40 minutes)

1. Pelvic and Hip Openers page 124, Fig. 24 A to D
2. Supported Bound Angle Pose page 128, Fig. 25
3. Supported Child's Pose page 140, Fig. 31
4. The Waterfall page 137, Fig. 30B
5. Revolved Belly Pose page 127, Fig. 24
6. Breathing Easy position page 141, Fig. 32
7. Choose one of the following breath inquiries:

   - Strengthening Diaphragmatic Breathing A or B page 149, Fig. 33A & B
   - Straw Breathing page 152, Fig. 34
   - The Three-Part Breath page 156
   - Alternate Nostril Breathing (try breathing in through the left nostril and out through the right nostril to cool the body) page 161, Fig. 35

Pain Relief

(Also see "Comeditation," listed under Resources. Comeditation is a breathing technique that has been used extensively for treating pain.)

The breath provides a natural massage to the entire body. This massage, in and of itself, is a pain reliever, signaling the nervous system that all is well. When we hold our breaths in response to pain or in the hope that this will eliminate the pain we actually increase the pain. What causes pain and the perpetuation of pain is often not the original sensation but our reaction to it and our imagining of what *might* happen if the pain continues or gets worse.

Many of my students have had long histories of back pain. This breathing technique has helped many of them to prevent a spasm from setting up shop in their backs, but you can use it for any kind of pain. Instead of tensing and giving in to fear when you feel the first sharp twinge of pain, quiet your mind and calm your breathing. Don't think about all the things that may happen if the pain increases. Instead begin to breathe into the area where you feel the sensations, and observe the sensations with as much detachment as you can muster as they arise over a period of minutes. By continuing to breathe rather than freezing or holding your breath, you may be able to diminish or completely abort a potential spasm or pain cycle. My back pain clients have said that even if their backs do spasm, it doesn't last as long nor is it as severe as previous episodes.

If you use this technique, it's important that you do not have an attachment to the outcome. If you do, the very tension and expectation may undermine your attempts to relax. Imagine that your breath is originating from the very center of where you feel the pain. Touch yourself with your breath with the utmost tenderness and compassion. It's not important for you to make a big, mechanical movement with your breathing, even the tiniest movement can have a profound effect in releasing tension.

Dr. Erik Peper at San Francisco State University has found the following techniques beneficial for pain sufferers:[12]

- **Exhale** *Exhale* whenever you *anticipate* a painful stimuli, whether the pain is caused by an injection or the drill of the dentist. Our natural tendency is to inhale and hold the breath. When we exhale we are saying, "I accept that this is going to happen" instead of flinching from our experience.

- **Pacing and Leading** If you are a health practitioner, friend, partner, or parent working with someone in pain, you can pace and lead them into a slower breathing rhythm simply by slowing down your own breathing (see comeditation for information on a very profound use for pacing and leading the breath). First observe how the other person is breathing and then gradually shift the way you are breathing, increasing your exhalation and being conscious of pausing at the end of the exhalation. I sometimes sigh as I exhale and encourage the other person to do so. As Dr. Peper contends, "Energy fields are contagious!"

- **Stroking** Pain in a specific area of the body is often accompanied by a diminishing awareness, so that we disown the painful part. By stroking lightly along the area that is painful the person begins to reconnect to that place in themselves. Breathing into the area increases. The stroking also feels very pleasurable and reassuring. If you are doing this with someone else make sure they are comfortable being touched this way.

- **Gasp Technique** If you are not sure whether breath work can help you control pain levels try this experiment. Exaggerate a gasp pattern of breathing (the kind of breathing you do when someone jumps out at you). If the pain increases in a specific area in your body it is very likely that breath retraining will be helpful in reducing the pain. This technique also may increase your confidence that you have some control over your pain—if you can make your pain worse through breathing badly, then you can make it better through breathing well.

The causes of pain are so diverse, from cancer and organic diseases to sports injuries, that no one practice program would cover all the possible bases. I encourage you to choose movements from chapter 5 that address your particular needs.

Do These Inquiries First

～ Inquiry: The Marriage of Breath and Movement (keep the movements very small) page 16, Fig. 1 & 2
～ Inquiry: Contracting Your Diaphragm page 73

Practice Sequence (20 minutes)

1. Pelvic and Hip Opener page 124, (Fig. 23A & B only)
2. Revolved Belly Pose page 127, Fig. 24
3. Effortless Rest position page 18, Fig. 3

Choose one from the following:
- Following the Lure of the Breath page 143
- Back Breathing (especially good for back pain) page 98, Fig. 16
- Organ Breathing (for pain of an organic source) page 100, Illustration 12
- The Three-Part Breath (excellent for letting go of the built-up tension that often accompanies chronic pain) page 156

Pre-performance Anxiety

Whether you are preparing to propose to your partner or presenting a financial report at the office, pre-performance anxiety can be quelled very successfully through simple breathing practices. The following techniques are quick and easy to use and can be done at any time in a sitting, standing, or reclining position.

Do These Inquiries First

∼ Inquiry: Contracting the Diaphragm page 73
∼ Inquiry: The Dance of the Diaphragms page 60, Illustrations 13 & 14

General Techniques Use what you learn from these inquiries to keep yourself calm both before and during your "performance."

∼ Inquiry: Back Breathing (alone) page 98, Fig. 16
∼ Inquiry: Lengthening the Exhalation page 102
∼ Inquiry: Soft Eyes/Open Diaphragm page 103

Specifics

1. Diaphragm Release B page 135
(If you are sitting in a public place you can do this release by leaning over the back of a chair with your arms behind your head.)
2. Chose one of the following:
   • Alternate Nostril Breathing (with counting) page 161, Fig. 35
   • The Three-Part Breath page 156

Post-Traumatic Stress

When we receive a sudden shock the diaphragm "jumps" in the chest and contracts. In most cases this deep contraction is a momentary event, but if we have been badly shaken up, such as after a car accident, it's quite common for hyperventilation and erratic breathing to continue for hours. If severe shock occurs over and over again, as was the case for many of our Vietnam veterans and also for survivors of horrific abuse or catastrophe, the initial shock can embed itself as a more permanent pattern in the nervous system. Then it is called Post-Traumatic Stress syndrome or disorder. If you believe you suffer from such shock, use the practice session that follows to help breakdown the holding pattern, and get professional help. The other techniques can be used at any time as your "first line of defense" helping you to cope with an immediate situation.

Breathing First Aid for Sudden Shock

1. Back Breathing (alone) page 98
2. Lengthening Your Exhalation page 102
3. The Three-Part Breath (do one or two cycles, exhaling through the mouth if this helps you to relax) page 156
4. Concentrate on the sensation of your feet on the ground. Imagine that you are breathing in through your legs. This shift of attention into the lower body can help ground the body and stop the panicking mind from going into a "full spin."

Practice Sequence (For more chronic conditions) (30 minutes)

1. Pelvic and Hip Openers page 124, (Fig. 23A & B only)
2. Revolved Belly Pose page 127, Fig. 24
3. Supported Child's Pose (very comforting for children) page 140, Fig. 31
4. The Waterfall (cover the eyes and forehead with an ace bandage wound *lightly* around the head) page 137, Fig. 30B
5. Assume the Effortless Rest position or the Breathing Easy position and choose one of the following to finish:
   • Lengthening the Exhalation (10 minutes) page 102
   • The Three-Part Breath (10 minutes) page 156

Quitting Smoking

When Dr. Tom Ferguson interviewed smokers for his book *The No-Nag, No-Guilt, Do-It-Yourself Guide to Quitting Smoking* (Ballantine, New York), he found that 84 percent of those interviewed would quit if they could do so without the unpleasant withdrawal symptoms. What was more interesting was that while withdrawal was considered a major reason for smokers to stay hooked, people felt that smoking provided them with some very positive benefits. High on the list of "benefits" was the belief that smoking helped them deal with stressful situations such as an overstimulating workplace or a painful, upsetting event. Although most of us non-smokers postulate that smokers puff because it makes them feel comfortable or even fashionably cool in social situations, this benefit ranked low on the list compared with the smoker's desire to use cigarettes to unwind and relax. While the smoker may use smoking to cope with life's inevitable pressures, the addiction of smoking creates its own tension as the body repeatedly signals for its regular hit of nicotine (which can be as often as every 20 minutes in the nicotine addict).

Considering that taking a "long drag" is in reality a lengthened breath cycle, it's not surprising that smokers feel so many benefits from smoking, including the perception that smoking helps them concentrate. Underneath the immediate alleviation of discomfort, many smokers use their habit to repress rather than deal with more deeply rooted feelings of anger or sadness. Because smoking is such a difficult habit to overcome, I recommend a threefold strategy. First, find out as much as you can about how to quit. Dr. Ferguson's book is an excellent way to start, and you may be able to attend a quit smoking program at a local clinic or through your health practitioner. Second, plan at least three "feel good" sessions for yourself each week using the general program I've outlined. This will help you let off steam and prevent the buildup of tension throughout the week. Third, cultivate "breathing breaks" instead of cigarette breaks. You can do this even before you attempt to quit smoking. When you feel the urge to smoke, take a moment to become quiet so that you can determine what is going on inside you and outside you. Can you identify the key stressor at that moment? It may be a specific event, such as an overdue work report, or it may be less specific, such as an unhappy relationship. And then try one of the strategies below for at least one minute.

Techniques

～ Inquiry: Back Breathing (alone) page 98
～ Inquiry: Lengthening the Exhalation page 102

1. Straw Breathing (if you are in a public place try breathing out through a cigarette holder—it will make you less conspicuous and give you the feeling of smoking.) page 152, Fig. 34
2. The Three-Part Breath page 156
3. Kapalabhati page 158

Sinusitis

Regular nasal irrigation, or *neti,* has been found remarkably effective for clearing up sinus infections. Refer to the section on nasal washes on page 62. Once you have irrigated the nasal passages, try Alternate Nostril Breathing. For palliative relief, especially if you are unable to breathe at night, try using Breathe Right® nasal strips (see Resources).

Resources

OTHER HELPFUL BOOKS ON BREATHING

Breathing for Health with Biofeedback
Erik Peper, Ph.D.
Thought Technology Ltd.
2180 Belgrave Ave.
Montreal, Quebec
Canada H4A 2L8
A booklet and two audiocassettes with excellent instructions for learning diaphragmatic breathing and relaxation skills. You can use the audios with or without the use of biofeedback devices.

Breath, Mind and Consciousness
Harish Johari
Destiny Books
Rochester, VT, 1989
An extremely comprehensive analysis of the effects of nostril dominance from a traditional yogic perspective.

Hyperventilation Syndrome: A Handbook for Bad Breathers
Dinah Bradley
Celestial Arts
Berkeley, CA, 1992
A short and snappy manual for people with hyperventilation syndrome, using lay persons' language and humorous illustrations.

Science of Breath
Swami Rama, Rudolph Ballentine, and Alan Hymes
Himalayan International Institute of Yoga Science and Philosophy
Honesdale, PA, 1981
An excellent little introduction to breathing with fascinating chapters on the anatomy of breathing.

The Perceptible Breath
Ilse Middendorf, 1990
Available through Somatic Resources (includes audiocassettes), P.O. Box 2067
Berkeley, CA 94702
(510) 540-7600
This book has some very interesting ideas but is unfortunately difficult to follow without the help of an instructor. You may wish to contact a Middendorf Instructor through:

The Middendorf Breath Institute
198 Mississippi
San Francisco, CA 94107
(415) 255-2174 or 255-2175

Ways to Better Breathing
Carola Speads
Healing Arts Press
Rochester, VT, 1992
Beautifully written with easy-to-follow breathing "experiments."

CLINICAL HELP FOR THOSE WITH BREATHING (AND OTHER) DISORDERS

Biofeedback training for those with breathing disorders
Biofeedback has been found particularly effective for those suffering from asthma, hypertension, hyperventilation, panic attacks and anxiety disorders as well as numerous other health problems such as chronic headaches and migraines. Almost all biofeedback practitioners incorporate the instruction of diaphragmatic breathing in their sessions. If you feel your problem warrants clinical supervision or do not feel confident to work on your own, you may want to seek out a licensed practitioner.
Contact:
The Association for Applied Psychophysiology and Biofeedback
10200 West 44th Ave., Suite 304
Wheat Ridge, CO 80033-2840
Include a SASE and they will send the name of a contact person in your area.

Comeditation: A breathing technique for those with life-threatening illness and their caregivers.
Tibetan physicians and priests have used "comeditation" or "cross breathing" for centuries
to help the dying enter a meditative state and stop the racing mind and terror that often
accompanies illness and death. Richard Boerstler and Hulen Kornfeld, two of the major
proponents of comeditation, have been teaching the technique at hospitals and medical
schools throughout the United States. The technique centers around guiding the patient
into slow, deep, and relaxed breathing using verbal cues together with sounds such as *ah*
paced with the client's exhalation. It's not reliant on having a particular religious or spiritual belief contends Boerstler, who works extensively with AIDS patients. The process
slows respiration and pulse rate, lowers body temperature and blood pressure, releases anxiety, and reduces pain. This technique can be used for those in chronic pain and those facing life-threatening illness. For information on how to learn the technique or hospitals that
employ comeditation contact:

Richard Boerstler, Learning Center for Supportive Care
14 Orchard Lane
Lincoln, MA 01773
(617) 259-8936 and (508) 394-6520
or
Associates in Thanatology
115 Blue Rock Rd.
South Yarmouth, MA 02664

There is also a new release by the founders:

Life to Death: Harmonizing the Transition
Richard W. Boerstler and Hulen S. Kornfeld
Inner Traditions
P.O. Box 388
Rochester, VT 05767
(800) 246-8648

PROPS FOR BREATH WORK

Hugger Mugger Yoga Products
31 W. Gregson Ave.
Salt Lake City, UT 84115
1-800-473-4888
They supply breathing bolsters, called *pranayama* bolsters, eye bags, and yoga blankets.

Yoga Props
3055 23rd Street-J
San Francisco, CA 94110
(415) 285-YOGA (9642)
They supply 10-lb. sandbags and a breathing bolster that is specifically shaped (30″ × 8″ × 3″) to support the back during reclined breathing practice. They also carry inexpensive wool-blend blankets that can be used to provide cushioning and warmth for relaxation work.

Living Arts
2434 Main St., 2nd Floor
Santa Monica, CA 90405
(800) 2-LIVING

Tools for Yoga
P.O. Box 99
Chatham, NJ 07928
(201) 966-5311

Fish Crane
P.O. Box 791029
New Orleans, LA 70179
(800) 959-6116

Essential Products Alliance, Ltd.
Narial Nasal Cup
200 Frankfort Street
Versailles, KY 40383
1-800-817-8740
They sell *neti* pots for nasal irrigation.

The Original Neti Pot
Himalayan Publishers Dept. YI
RR 1, Box 405
Honesdale, PA 18431
1-800-822-4547
Suppliers of *neti* pots for nose cleansing.

Nasal Dilators
Nasal adhesive strips consist of a small adhesive bandage strip that is placed across the nose (halfway between the bridge and the end of the nose). As the flexible strip attempts to

spring back to a flat shape it gently opens the nasal passage way, allowing you to breathe easier. The producers of one brand, Breathe Right®, claim that this product reduces nasal airway resistance by "an average of 31%, a resistance reduction comparable to many over-the-counter nasal sprays." Consumer reaction appears to be extremely positive as those with chronic allergies, nighttime congestion, and structural problems such as a deviated septum consider it an exciting alternative to taking chemical medications. Athletes have also found the product very good for opening the breathing passages during exercise. One drawback is their price: I paid almost $6.00 for ten strips. A good night's sleep and freedom from medications that cause drowsiness and other side effects, however, may well be worth the price. They are available in any well-stocked drugstore.

MEDITATION AND MINDFULNESS BOOKS AND CENTERS

BOOKS:

Being Peace
Thich Nhat Hanh
Parallax Press
Berkeley, CA, 1987

The Miracle of Mindfulness: A Manual for Meditation
Thich Nhat Hanh
Beacon Press
Boston, MA, 1976

A Path with Heart: A Guide Through the Perils and Promises of Spiritual Life
Jack Kornfield
Bantam Books, 1993

Wherever You Go, There You Are: Mindfulness Meditation in Everyday Life
Jon Kabat-Zinn
Hyperion, 1994

BOOKS ON YOGA:

Yoga for Body, Breath, and Mind
A. G. Mohan
Rudra Press, Cambridge, MA, and
International Association of Yoga Therapists, Los Angeles, CA, 1993
Basic practice routines with breathing guidelines.

The Runner's Yoga Book: A Balanced Approach to Fitness
Jean Couch
Rodmell Press
Berkeley, CA, 1990
A simple, no-nonsense guide to basic yoga postures for athlete and non-athlete alike.

Relax and Renew: Restful Yoga for Stressful Times
Judith Lasater, Ph.D., P.T.
Rodmell Press
Berkeley, CA, 1995
Restorative yoga postures for stressful times. Special sections on practice during menstruation, menopause, and pregnancy, and for those with back pain.

Yoga for Pregnancy
Sandra Jordan
St. Martin's Press
New York, NY 1989
A simple guide for safe yoga practice during and after pregnancy.

YOGA TEACHER DIRECTORIES

Yoga Journal Magazine
2054 University Ave.
Berkeley, CA 94704
(510) 841-9200
Fax: (510) 644-3101
A special supplement updated annually in the July/August issue of the *Yoga Journal*.

Yoga International's Guide to Yoga Teachers and Classes
R.R. 1, Box 407
Honesdale, PA 18431
(800) 821-YOGA
This listing is updated annually as a supplement to the January/February issue of *Yoga International* magazine.

"The Breathing Body" seminars
Conducted by Donna Farhi, R.M.T., these seminars are open to individuals, teachers, body workers, and health care professionals. For more information contact: The Hatha Yoga School of Sumner, 42 Nayland St. Christchurch 8, New Zealand. Fax: (03) 326-5257.

Notes

CHAPTER ONE

1. Drug-Free Relief for Pregnancy Headaches," *American Health,* 15 (June 1995):26. Researchers at the University of Pittsburgh Medical Center found that pregnant women who had previously used drugs to control chronic tension or migraine headaches reported fewer or less intense headaches after four treatment sessions, using deep breathing, biofeedback, and stretching and strengthening exercises. Most did not return to medication after childbirth and reported the same results at home without biofeedback devices.
2. P. Luna-Massey, and E. Peper, "Clinical observation on breath patterns and pain relief in chronic pain patients," *Proceedings of the Seventeenth Annual Meeting of The Association for Applied Psychophysiology and Biofeedback* (Wheat Ridge, Colo.: BSA, 1986):82–84.
3. S. Fahrion, et al., "Biobehavioral treatment of essential hypertension: A group outcome study," *Biofeedback and Self-Regulation* 11 (1986):257–78.
4. Robert Fried, Ph.D., *The Breath Connection* (New York: Plenum Press, 1990).
5. Support for asthma treatment comes from the following sources: R. Fried, *The Hyperventilation Syndrome* (Baltimore: The Johns Hopkins University Press, 1987); M. K. Tandon, "Adjunct Treatment with Yoga in Chronic Severe Airways Obstruction," *Thorax,* 33 (1978):514–17. Their study showed yoga improved exercise tolerance in asthma patients and reduced their need for medical intervention; R. Nagarantha, and H. R. Nagendra, "Yoga for Bronchial Asthma: A Controlled Study," *British Medical Journal,* 291 (October 19, 1985). They demonstrated that asthma sufferers who practiced sixty-minute daily yoga regimens of breathing exercises, postures, and mediation experienced significantly fewer asthma attacks, had greater lung capacity, and had less need for medication; Dan C. Stanescu, et al., "Pattern of Breathing and Ventilatory Response to CO_2 in Subjects Practicing Hatha Yoga," *Journal of Applied Physiology,* Dec. 1981; E. Peper, and V. Tibbetts, "Fifteen-month follow up with asthmatics utilizing EMG/incentive inspirometer feedback," *Biofeedback and Self Regulation* 17 (2) (1992):143–51.

6. L. C. Lum, "The syndrome of habitual chronic hyperventilation," in V. Hill, ed., *Modern Trends in Psychosomatic Medicine* (London: Butterworth, 1976):196–230.

7. J. Van Dixhoorn, *Relaxation Therapy in Cardiac Rehabilitation* (Den Haag: Doninklijke Bibliotheek, 1990).

8. R.R. Freedman, and S. Woodward, "Behavioral treatment of menopausal hot flushes: evaluation by ambulatory monitoring," *American Journal of Obstetrics and Gynecology,* 167 (2) (1992):257–78.

9. L. M. Germaine, and R.R. Freedman, "Behavioral treatment of menopausal flashes: evaluation by objective methods." *Journal of Consulting Clinical Psychology,* 52 (1984):1,072–79.

10. O. Miller, "A Sharing of Breaths," *Yoga Journal* (March/April 1993):136.

11. P.B.F. Nixon, "Human Functions and the Heart," in D. Seedhouse, and A. Cribb, eds., *Changing Ideas in Health Care* (New York: John Wiley & Sons, 1989):37.

CHAPTER TWO

1. This exercise was adapted from *The Perceptible Breath* by Ilse Middendorf. While the author is familiar with Ms. Middendorf's work she does not purport to practice or teach the Middendorf method.

2. E. Peper, "Comparison of Diaphragmatic Training Methods," *Proceedings of the Twenty-Fifth Annual Meeting of The Association for Applied Psychophysiology and Biofeedback* (Wheat Ridge, Colo: AAPB, 1994).

3. E. Peper, and V. Tibbetts, "Effects of Paced Breathing on Inhalation Volumes," *Proceedings of the Twenty-First Annual Meeting of The Association for Applied Psychophysiology and Biofeedback* (Wheat Ridge, Colo.: AAPB, 1990):157–59.

CHAPTER THREE

1. This idea was presented to me by Bonnie Bainbridge Cohen at a workshop on "The Dynamics of Breathing," San Francisco, Calif., 1994.

2. E. Peper, and V. Tibbetts, "Enhanced stability with diaphragmatic breathing: Avoid stumbling due to chest breathing," *Proceedings of the Twenty-Fourth Annual Meeting of the Association for Applied Psychophysiology and Biofeedback* (Wheat Ridge, Colo.: AAPB, 1993):222–24.

3. Dinah Bradley, *Hyperventilation Syndrome: A Handbook for Bad Breathers* (Berkeley, Calif.: Celestial Arts, 1991). Bradley notes that 30 to 40 percent of suspected heart attack victims showing up for care at emergency and coronary care units were subsequently found to have absolutely nothing wrong with their hearts.

4. J. Van Dixhoorn, *Relaxation Therapy in Cardiac Rehabilitation* (Den Haag: Doninklijke Bibliotheek, 1990).

5. A. Hymes, and P. Nuernberger, "Breathing Patterns Found in Heart Attack Patients," *Research Bulletin of the Himalayan International Institute* 2 (2)(1980):10–12. The authors found that the primary or habitual breathing pattern of all 153 patients in a coronary care unit of a large hospital was thoracic.

6. James Funderburk, Ph.D., "Science of Breath," *Science Studies Yoga* (Honesdale, Penn.: Himalayan Institute, 1977):36–413.

7. Andrew P. Thomas, "Yoga and Cardiovascular Function," *Journal of the International Association of Yoga Therapists,* 4:39–41.

8. Robert Fried, Ph.D., *The Breath Connection* (New York: Plenum Press, 1990), 62.

9. The following present supporting evidence of nostril dominance and its effect on the nervous system: Ernest Lawrence Rossi, Ph.D., with David Nimmons, *The Twenty Minute Break: Using the New Science of Ultradian Rhythms* (Los Angeles: Jeremy Tarcher, Inc., 1991); and David Shannahoff-Khalsa, "Lateralized Rhythms of the Central and Autonomic Nervous System," *International Journal of Psychophysiology,* 11 (issue 3) (1991):222–51.

10. Essential Products Alliance was helpful in providing comprehensive material on the health benefits and correct use of nasal irrigation. See Resources for information on nasal irrigation products.

CHAPTER FOUR

1. V. Tibbetts, and E. Peper, "Effects of Imagery and Position on Breathing Patterns," *Proceedings of the Twenty-Seventh Annual Meeting of The Association for Applied Psychophysiology and Biofeedback* (Wheat Ridge, Colo.: AAPB, 1996). In addition, these researchers found that bracing and respiration patterns could also be altered by *imagining* walking on a hard or soft surface. That is, one could increase or reduce the arousal response by imagining walking on a soft meadow or walking on a hard concrete surface.

2. Conversations with Dr. Erik Peper, San Francisco State University, May 18, 1995.

3. E. Peper, and V. Tibbetts, "Effects of Paced Breathing on Inhalation Volumes," *Proceedings of the Twenty-First Annual Meeting of The Association for Applied Psychophysiology and Biofeedback* (Wheat Ridge, Colo.: AAPB, 1990):157–59.

4. E. Peper, et al., "Repetitive Strain Injury: Prevent Computer User Injury With Biofeedback: Assessment and Training Protocol," *Electromyography Thought Technology,* 1994.

   This study showed that without kinesthetic awareness and without the skills to reduce tension, ergonomic adjustments with intermittent rest periods are not sufficient to reduce the risk of injury, especially repetitive strain injury (*RSI*) to computer users. That is, even with ideal work conditions, computer workers seem to brace inappropriately and excessively, accompanied by an increased rate of respiration and chest breathing. With training in kinesthetic awareness, computer users can change these unconscious habits.

5. Robert Fried, Ph.D., *The Breath Connection* (New York: Plenum Press, 1990).

6. Carola Speads, *Ways to Better Breathing* (Rochester, Vermont: Healing Arts Press, 1992).

CHAPTER SIX

1. The following have found evidence of meditation decreasing sensitivity to carbon dioxide: R. Jevning, R. K. Wallace, and M. Beidebach, "The Physiology of Meditation: A Review. A Wakeful Hypometabolic Integrated Response," in *Neuroscience and Biobehavioral Reviews,* 16 (1992):415–24; and N. Wolkove, et al., "Effect of Transcendental Meditation on Breathing and Respiratory Control," *Journal of Applied Physiology* 56 (1984):607–12.

2. This exercise is adapted from Carola Speads, *Ways to Better Breathing* (Rochester, Vermont: Healing Arts Press), 1992.

3. Janet King, M.D., Michael R. Bye, M.D., and James Demopoulos, M.D., "Exercise Programs for Asthmatic Children," in *Comprehensive Therapy* (November 1984); and S. B. Kleinberg, *Educating the Chronically Ill Child* (Rockville, Md.: Aspen Systems, 1982):90.
4. Adapted from "Knocking at the Gate of Life" and other healing exercises from Edward Chang, Ph.D., *Official Manual of the People's Republic of China* (Emmaus, Penn.:Rodale Press, 1985).

CHAPTER SEVEN

1. Ruthy Alon, *Mindful Spontaneity* (New York: Avery Publishing, 1990).

CHAPTER EIGHT

1. Alix Kates Shulman, *Drinking the Rain* (New York: Farrar, Straus & Giroux, 1995).
2. Richard Miller, "Breath of Life," *Yoga Journal* (September/October 1994).

PRACTICE GUIDES

1. Carola Speads, *Ways to Better Breathing* (Rochester, Vermont: Healing Arts Press, 1992).
2. John R. M. Goyeche, Ph.D. et al., "Asthma: The Yoga Perspective, Part II: Yoga Therapy in the Treatment of Asthma," *Journal of Asthma Research,* 19 (3) (1982):189–201.
3. John R. M. Goyeche, Ph.D. et al., "Asthma: The Yoga Perspective Part I, The Somatopsychic Imbalance in Asthma: Towards a Holistic Therapy," *Journal of Asthma Research,* 17 (3) (April 1980).
4. The following studied deep breathing combined with yoga and meditation, and its impact on various ailments: M. K. Tandon, "Adjunct Treatment with Yoga in Chronic Severe Airways Obstruction," *Thorax,* 33 (1978):514–17; R. Nagarantha, and H. R. Nagendra, "Yoga for Bronchial Asthma: A Controlled Study," *British Medical Journal,* 291, (October 19, 1985); and Dan C. Stanescu, et al., "Pattern of Breathing and Ventilatory Response to CO_2 in Subjects Practicing Hatha Yoga," *Journal of Applied Physiology* (December 1981).
5. Carl Jones, *Alternative Birth* (Los Angeles: Jeremy Tarcher Inc., 1991).
6. Chloe Fisher, "The Management of Labor: A Midwife's View," in *Episiotomy and the Second Stage of Labor,* Sheila Kitzinger and Penny Simkin, eds. (Seattle: Pennypress, 1984):57.
7. Constance Beynon, "The Normal Second Stage of Labour. A Plea for Reform in Its Conduct," *Journal of Obstetrics and Gynecology of the British Empire,* 64 (6) (December 1957).
8. Rahima Baldwin, *Special Delivery* (Millbrae, Calif.: Les Femmes, 1979).
9. Penny Simkin, "Active and Physiologic Management of Second Stage: A Review and Hypothesis," in *Episiotomy and Second Stage of Labor,* Sheila Kitzinger and Penny Simkin, eds. (Seattle: Pennypress, 1984):7.
10. Duncan Mackay, "The Human Machine Shatters Pain Barrier," *The Press,* Christchurch, New Zealand, July 21, 1995.
11. E. Peper, and J. Clavenna, "Correction of a Dysfunctional Respiratory Pattern in Freestyle Swimming: A Case Report," *Proceedings of the Twenty-Fourth Annual Meeting of the Association for Applied Psychophysiology and Biofeedback* (Wheat Ridge, Colo.: AAPB, 1993).
12. Conversations with Professor Erik Peper, San Francisco State University, July 1995.

Acknowledgments

I feel an enormous appreciation for all my friends and family who have so generously given their support to this project. In particular, my loving partner, Mark Bouckoms, who reminded me to take a daily walk by the sea and kept the fire going in more ways than one during the cold winter months of writing. To my mother Louise and stepfather Jack, who in combination have been a familial fan club, cheering on my efforts. This book would have never come to fruition were it not for my literary agent, Laurie Fox, and my editor, Bryan Oettel, whose kindness and boundless enthusiasm have bolstered my confidence throughout the project. My special thanks to Dr. Erik Peper for his generous interviews and for sending me scientific papers and research material that would have been difficult to procure in New Zealand. Thanks also to Dr. Roger Cole, Jane Campbell-Kaye, and Peter Coates for reviewing specific sections of the text and providing me with helpful research material. To Stephen Crowe, who stretched himself beyond the call of duty to produce the beautiful illustrations for the book. To Fred and Amanda Stimson, for taking such great care in producing the photographs for this book, not to mention the fabulous lunches during the long photo shoot. Special thanks to Carol Banquer and Dave and Dione King, who have provided me with a peaceful sanctuary in San Francisco during my teaching tours and research stays and who have been extraordinary friends through thick and thin. Finally, thank you to all the teachers who inspired me to follow my own excitement, to the yoga centers and individuals that have supported my teaching visits, and to the hundreds of yoga students who opened themselves to the breath and through their participation helped me to formulate the core material for this book.

Grateful acknowledgment is made for the permission to reprint from the following:

Jane Huang, in collaboration with Michael Wurmbrand, *The Primordial Breath*, vol. 1 (Torrance, Calif.: Original Books, Inc., 1990), pages 11–12, 39, 45.

Jordan Fisher-Smith, "Field Observations: An Interview with Wendell Berry," in *The Sun: A Magazine of Ideas* (February 1994), page 10.

Coleman Barks, *Rumi, We are Three* (Athens, Ga: Maypop Books, 1987), page 27.

Luther Standing Bear, *Land of the Spotted Eagle* (Lincoln: University of Nebraska Press, 1978). Copyright renewal by May Jones, 1960, page 250.

Excerpted Avavnuk/Eskimo poem from *Intellectual Life of the Iglulik Eskimos* by Knut Rasmussen, translated from Danish by W. E. Calver, 1930. Reprinted in *Every Part of this Earth is Sacred,* edited by Jana Stone (San Francisco: Harper San Francisco, 1993), page 123.

Reprinted from "Yoga and Cardiovascular Function" by Dr. Andrew Thomas, *Journal of the International Association of Yoga Therapists,* vol. 4, 1993, page 40.

Bonnie Bainbridge Cohen, *Sensing, Feeling and Action* (Northampton, Mass.: Contact Editions, 1993), page 17.

Archie Fire Lame Deer and Richard Erdoes, *Gift of Power* (Sante Fe, N.M.: Bear & Co., 1992), page 180.

Adapted from Robert Fried, *The Breath Connection* (New York: Insight Books, 1990), pages 173–175.

Robert Bly, *The Kabir Book,* © 1971, 1977 by Robert Bly. Reprinted by permission of Beacon Press, page 33.

David Whyte, *Where Many Rivers Meet* (Langley, Wash.: Many Rivers Press, 1990).

Carola Speads, *Ways to Better Breathing* (Rochester, Vt.: Healing Arts Press, 1992), page 12.

William Kotzwinkle, "Jewel of the Moon," from *Yellow Silk: Erotic Arts and Letters,* edited by Lily Pond and Richard Russo. (New York: Harmony Books, 1990), page 60.

Alix Kates Shulman, *Drinking the Rain* (New York: Farrar, Strauss & Giroux, 1995), pages 53–54.

Sharon Gladden, "In Rain," in *MoonJuice IV* (Santa Cruz, Calif.: Embers Press, 1981), page 67.

Robert Bly, "A Man and a Woman Sit Near Each Other," in *Loving a Woman in Two Worlds* (New York: Doubleday, 1986).

Ruthy Alon, "Movement for Life, Movement for Love," in *Mindful Spontaneity* (Dorset, England: Prism Press, 1990), chap. 4.

Excerpted from *Being Peace* by Thich Nhat Hanh (Berkeley, Calif.: Parallax Press, 1987), page 5.

Special thanks go to Essential Products Alliance, Inc. for providing information on nasal irrigation.